Adult Acquired Flatfoot Deformity

Editors

ALAN R. CATANZARITI
ROBERT W. MENDICINO

CLINICS IN PODIATRIC
MEDICINE AND SURGERY

www.podiatric.theclinics.com

Consulting Editor
THOMAS ZGONIS

July 2014 • Volume 31 • Number 3

ELSEVIER

1600 John F. Kennedy Boulevard • Suite 1800 • Philadelphia, Pennsylvania, 19103-2899

http://www.theclinics.com

CLINICS IN PODIATRIC MEDICINE AND SURGERY Volume 31, Number 3
July 2014 ISSN 0891-8422, ISBN-13: 978-0-323-31170-0

Editor: Jennifer Flynn-Briggs
Developmental Editor: Casey Jackson

Clinics in Podiatric Medicine and Surgery (ISSN 0891-8422) is published quarterly by Elsevier Inc., 360 Park Avenue South, New York, NY 10010-1710. Months of issue are January, April, July, and October. Business and Editorial Offices: 1600 John F. Kennedy Blvd., Ste. 1800, Philadelphia, PA 19103-2899. Customer Service Office: 3251 Riverport Lane, Maryland Heights, MO 63043. Periodicals postage paid at NewYork, NY and additional mailing offices. Subscription prices are $305.00 per year for US individuals, $450.00 per year for US institutions, $155.00 per year for US students and residents, $370.00 per year for Canadian individuals, $544.00 for Canadian institutions, $435.00 for international individuals, $544.00 per year for international institutions and $220.00 per year for Canadian and foreign students/residents. To receive student/resident rate, orders must be accompanied by name of affiliated institution, date of term, and the *signature* of program/residency coordinator on institution letterhead. Orders will be billed at individual rate until proof of status is received. Foreign air speed delivery is included in all *Clinics* subscription prices. All prices are subject to change without notice. POSTMASTER: Send address changes to *Clinics in Podiatric Medicine and Surgery*, Elsevier Health Sciences Division, Subscription Customer Service, 3251 Riverport Lane, Maryland Heights, MO 63043. **Customer Service: 1-800-654-2452 (US). From outside of the US, call 314-447-8871. Fax: 314-447-8029. E-mail: JournalsCustomerService-usa@elsevier.com (for print support); JournalsOnlineSupport-usa@elsevier.com (for online support).**

Reprints. For copies of 100 or more of articles in this publication, please contact the Commercial Reprints Department, Elsevier Inc., 360 Park Avenue South, New York, NY 10010-1710. Tel.: 212-633-3874; Fax: 212-633-3820; E-mail: reprints@elsevier.com.

Clinics in Podiatric Medicine and Surgery is covered in *MEDLINE/PubMed (Index Medicus)* and *EMBASE/Excerpta Medica*.

Contributors

CONSULTING EDITOR

THOMAS ZGONIS, DPM, FACFAS
Associate Professor and Director of Externship and Reconstructive Foot and Ankle Fellowship Programs, Division of Podiatric Medicine and Surgery, Department of Orthopaedic Surgery, University of Texas Health Science Center San Antonio, San Antonio, Texas

EDITORS

ALAN R. CATANZARITI, DPM, FACFAS
Director of Residency Training Program, Division of Foot and Ankle Surgery, West Penn Hospital, Allegheny Health Network, Pittsburgh, Pennsylvania

ROBERT W. MENDICINO, DPM, FACFAS
Foot and Ankle Surgeon, OhioHealth Orthopedic Surgeons, Department of Orthopoedics, Hilliard, Ohio; Faculty, Foot & Ankle Surgical Residency, West Penn Hospital, Pittsburgh, Pennsylvania

AUTHORS

ADEBOLA T. ADELEKE, DPM
Surgical Resident, Division of Foot & Ankle Surgery, West Penn Hospital, Pittsburgh, Pennsylvania

JOHN M. BACA, DPM
Surgical Resident, Division of Foot & Ankle Surgery, West Penn Hospital, Pittsburgh, Pennsylvania

ALAN R. CATANZARITI, DPM, FACFAS
Director of Residency Training Program, Division of Foot and Ankle Surgery, West Penn Hospital, Allegheny Health Network, Pittsburgh, Pennsylvania

JAMES M. COTTOM, DPM, FACFAS
Fellowship Director, Attending Physician, Coastal Orthopedics and Sports Medicine, Bradenton, Florida

RICHARD DERNER, DPM, FACFAS
Private Practice, Associated Foot and Ankle Centers of Northern Virginia, Lake Ridge, Virginia

LAWRENCE A. DIDOMENICO, DPM, FACFAS
Ankle and Foot Care Centers, Youngstown, Ohio; Adjunct Professor, Kent State University College of Podiatric Medicine; Section Director, St. Elizabeth Hospital, Youngstown, Ohio; Director of Reconstructive Rearfoot and Ankle Surgical Fellowship; Faculty, Heritage Valley Hospital, Beaver, Pennsylvania

BRIAN T. DIX, DPM
Surgical Resident, Division of Foot & Ankle Surgery, West Penn Hospital, Pittsburgh, Pennsylvania

ERICA L. EVANS, DPM
Foot & Ankle Institute, Foot & Ankle Surgery, West Penn Hospital, Pittsburgh, Pennsylvania

RAMY FAHIM, DPM, AACFAS
Fellow, Reconstructive Rearfoot and Ankle Surgical Fellowship, Ankle and Foot Centers, Youngstown, Ohio

MATTHEW J. HENTGES, DPM
Surgical Resident, Division of Foot and Ankle Surgery, West Penn Hospital, Allegheny Health Network, Pittsburgh, Pennsylvania

CHRISTOPHER F. HYER, DPM, MS, FACFAS
Fellowship Director, Attending Physician, Orthopedic Foot and Ankle Center, Westerville, Ohio

JARED M. MAKER, DPM, AACFAS
Fellow, Foot and Ankle Surgical Fellowship, Coastal Orthopedics and Sports Medicine, Bradenton, Florida

ROGER MARZANO, CPO, Cped
Yanke Bionics Clinics, Inc, Akron, Ohio

ROBERT W. MENDICINO, DPM, FACFAS
Foot and Ankle Surgeon, OhioHealth Orthopedic Surgeons, Department of Orthopoedics, Hilliard, Ohio; Faculty, Foot & Ankle Surgical Residency, West Penn Hospital, Pittsburgh, Pennsylvania

SAMUEL S. MENDICINO, DPM, FACFAS
Director, West Houston Medical and Surgical Residency Program PMSR/RRA, West Houston Medical Center, Houston, Texas

KYLE R. MOORE, DPM
Surgical Resident, Division of Foot and Ankle Surgery, West Penn Hospital, Allegheny Health Network, Pittsburgh, Pennsylvania

KYLE S. PETERSON, DPM, AACFAS
Fellow, Advanced Foot and Ankle Surgical Fellowship, Orthopedic Foot and Ankle Center, Westerville, Ohio

PHILLIP E. RICHARDSON, DPM
Surgical Resident, Division of Foot & Ankle Surgery, West Penn Hospital, Pittsburgh, Pennsylvania

ZACHARY M. THOMAS, DPM
PGYIII, Heritage Valley Hospital, Beaver, Pennsylvania

JEREMY L. WALTERS, DPM
West Houston Medical and Surgical Residency Program PMSR/RRA, West Houston Medical Center, Houston, Texas

COLIN ZDENEK, DPM
Surgical Resident, Division of Foot & Ankle Surgery, West Penn Hospital, Pittsburgh, Pennsylvania

Contents

and soft tissue abnormalities visible on plain radiographs, ultrasound, and magnetic resonance imaging. Imaging abnormalities include various combinations of malalignment, anatomic variants, and enthesopathic and tendinopathic changes. A thorough understanding of differences between anatomic and pathologic presentations of structures in various imaging modalities is an essential tool for clinical and surgical planning.

Adult acquired flatfoot represents a spectrum of deformities affecting the foot and the ankle. The flexible, or nonfixed, deformity must be treated appropriately to decrease the morbidity that accompanies the fixed flatfoot deformity or when deformity occurs in the ankle joint. A comprehensive approach must be taken, including addressing equinus deformity, hindfoot valgus, forefoot supinatus, and medial column instability. A combination of osteotomies, limited arthrodesis, and medial column stabilization procedures are required to completely address the deformity.

Adult acquired flatfoot deformity is a progressive disorder with multiple symptoms and degrees of deformity. Stage II adult acquired flatfoot can be divided into stage IIA and IIB based on severity of deformity. Surgical procedures should be chosen based on severity as well as location of the flatfoot deformity. Care must be taken not to overcorrect the flatfoot deformity so as to decrease the possibility of lateral column overload as well as stiffness.

The clinical presentation of adult flatfoot can range from a flexible deformity with normal joint integrity to a rigid, arthritic flat foot. Debate still exists regarding the surgical management of stage II deformities, especially in the presence of medial column instability. This article reviews and discusses various surgical options for the correction of stage II flatfoot reconstructive procedures. The authors discuss their opinion that is not always necessary to transfer the flexor digitorum longus tendon to provide relief and stability in this patient population. The anatomy, diagnosis, and current treatments of flexible flatfoot deformity are discussed.

The supination of the forefoot that develops with adult acquired flatfoot is defined as forefoot supinatus. This deformity is an acquired soft tissue adaptation in which the forefoot is inverted on the rearfoot. Forefoot supinatus can mimic and often be mistaken for a forefoot varus. A forefoot varus differs from forefoot supinatus in that a forefoot varus is a congenital osseous deformity that induces subtalar joint pronation, whereas forefoot supinatus is acquired and develops because of subtalar joint pronation. This article discusses the acquired form of forefoot supinatus.

The primary goal of triple arthrodesis for stage III and IV adult acquired flatfoot is to obtain a well-aligned plantigrade foot that will support the ankle in optimal alignment. Ancillary procedures including posterior muscle group lengthening, medial displacement calcaneal osteotomy, medial column stabilization, peroneus brevis tenotomy, or transfer and harvest of regional bone graft are often necessary to achieve adequate realignment. Image intensification is helpful in confirming optimal realignment before fixation. Results of triple arthrodesis are enhanced with adequate preparation of joint surfaces, bone graft/orthobiologics, 2-point fixation of all 3 tritarsal joints, and a vertical heel position.

Triple arthrodesis has traditionally been the procedure of choice for endstage adult-acquired flatfoot. The results have been universally good, and it has proven to be dependable and predictable. Nonetheless, complications have been reported following triple arthrodesis in certain patients. Selective arthrodesis of the talonavicular joint and subtalar joint through a single medial approach has been developed as an alternative. The authors especially prefer this procedure with severe transverse plane deformity and often choose this approach as an alternative to triple arthrodesis in high-risk patients, including those patients with diabetes mellitus, rheumatoid arthritis, long-term steroid use, and the elderly.

Adult acquired flatfoot deformity is a debilitating musculoskeletal condition affecting the lower extremity. Posterior tibial tendon dysfunction (PTTD) is the primary etiology for the development of a flatfoot deformity in an adult. PTTD is classified into 4 stages (with stage IV subdivided into stage IV-A and IV-B). This classification is described in detail in this article.

CLINICS IN PODIATRIC
MEDICINE AND SURGERY

FORTHCOMING ISSUES

October 2014
**Lower Extremity Complex
Trauma and Complications**
John J. Stapleton, *Editor*

January 2015
**Current Update on Orthobiologics
in Foot and Ankle Surgery**
Barry I. Rosenblum, *Editor*

RECENT ISSUES

April 2014
Hallux Abducto Valgus Surgery
Bob Baravarian, *Editor*

January 2014
**Medical and Surgical Management
of the Diabetic Foot and Ankle**
Peter A. Blume, DPM, FACFAS, *Editor*

October 2013
Pediatric Foot Deformities
Patrick DeHeer, *Editor*

RELATED ISSUE

Medical Clinics of North America
March 2014 (Volume 98, Issue 2, Pages 291–299)
Office-Based Management of Adult-Acquired Flatfoot Deformity, 19 December 2013
Sara Lyn Miniaci-Coxhead and Adolph Samuel Flemister, *Editors*

**DOWNLOAD
Free App!**

Review Articles
THE CLINICS

NOW AVAILABLE FOR YOUR iPhone and iPad

Foreword

Adult-Acquired Flatfoot Deformity

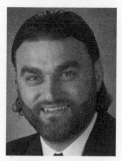

Thomas Zgonis, DPM, FACFAS
Consulting Editor

This edition of *Clinics in Podiatric Medicine and Surgery* is focused on the conservative and surgical treatment options of the adult-acquired flatfoot deformity. Recent technological advances in internal and external fixation products have provided surgeons with more stable constructs in addressing the multilevel adult-acquired flatfoot deformity. Surgical reconstructive options may vary from a medial column arthrodesis to a double, triple, or pantalar arthrodesis in the most severe cases. In the early stages of the deformity, tendinous versus combined osteotomy (medial calcaneal displacement osteotomy, lateral column lengthening, double calcaneal osteotomy), arthrodesis, and/or tendinous procedures may be performed according to the location and plane of deformity. Equal attention is given to the surgical correction of coexisting equinus deformities at the time of reconstruction.

This issue also reviews the most common conservative treatment options for this deformity, including bracing and ankle foot orthosis, and revisits the medical imaging studies in addressing the soft tissue and/or osseous pathologies related to the adult-acquired flatfoot deformity. The guest editors, Drs Alan R. Catanzariti and Robert W. Mendicino, along with the invited authors have done an excellent job in reviewing this progressive and debilitating pathologic entity that can be used as a great reference

Clin Podiatr Med Surg 31 (2014) xi–xii
http://dx.doi.org/10.1016/j.cpm.2014.05.001
0891-8422/14/$ – see front matter © 2014 Elsevier Inc. All rights reserved.

to our readers. I thank you again for your efforts and continuous contributions to *Clinics in Podiatric Medicine and Surgery.*

Thomas Zgonis, DPM, FACFAS
Division of Podiatric Medicine and Surgery
Department of Orthopaedic Surgery
University of Texas Health Science Center San Antonio
7703 Floyd Curl Drive, MSC 7776
San Antonio, TX 78229, USA

E-mail address:
zgonis@uthscsa.edu

Preface

Adult Acquired Flatfoot Deformity

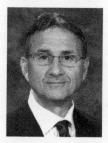 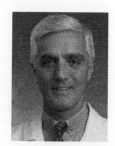

Alan R. Catanzariti, DPM, FACFAS   Robert W. Mendicino, DPM, FACFAS
Editors

The adult-acquired flatfoot deformity has remained one of the hottest topics in foot and ankle surgery for over two decades. In the 1980s, we began to see literature on the topic describing the pathologic abnormality and treatment options. As time passed, we began to see the evolution of surgical procedures ranging from a variety of soft tissue and tendinous augmentation to osseous procedures, including osteotomies and arthrodesing techniques. We also began to see a variety of classifications, MRI studies, and recommendations on surgical intervention based on imaging. Early on, patients were clumped into "cookie-cutter" subsets, and procedures were chosen on the soft tissue injury versus a combination of patient signs, symptoms, structure, and function of the affected limb.

Today, the clinician individualizes the plan for each patient by assessing all aspects of the patient's medical conditions, deformity, imaging, and function of the involved limb or limbs. Preoperative gait training and postoperative rehabilitation are also considered and discussed so that each individual has a thorough understanding of what is being considered and what the expectations are. The days of performing advanced imaging on each patient are gone. For a period of time, surgery was considered for nearly everyone but that too has changed.

Procedure selection and location remain regional considerations, but alignment has become standardized. The goal is to provide pain relief, eliminate progression of the deformity, and give an individual a sound structure with which to ambulate.

The following text should help the clinician understand the current evaluation and treatment recommendations while stimulating further academic discussion and research. We only hope that the next twenty or thirty years will see the same significant changes with care of this entity as we have in the past. Outcomes, nonoperative and

Clin Podiatr Med Surg 31 (2014) xiii–xiv
http://dx.doi.org/10.1016/j.cpm.2014.04.002
0891-8422/14/$ – see front matter © 2014 Elsevier Inc. All rights reserved.

operative techniques, fixation constructs, tissue augmentation, and bone growth will also improve as technology continues to advance.

Alan R. Catanzariti, DPM, FACFAS
Allegheny Health System
4800 Friendship Avenue, North Tower, First Floor
Pittsburgh, PA 15213, USA

Robert W. Mendicino, DPM, FACFAS
OhioHealth Orthopedic Surgeons
4343 All Seasons Drive, Suite 140
Hilliard, OH 43026, USA

E-mail addresses:
acatanzariti@faiwp.com (A.R. Catanzariti)
rmendicino@faiwp.com (R.W. Mendicino)

The Flexible Adult Flatfoot
Anatomy and Pathomechanics

Jeremy L. Walters, DPM*, Samuel S. Mendicino, DPM

KEYWORDS

- PTTD • Pes planus • Johnson and Strom • Posterior tibial • Tendon dysfunction
- Ankle

KEY POINTS

- Flexible flatfoot deformity in adults is a complex, multifaceted pathology.
- Understanding of the pertinent anatomy of flexible flatfoot deformity is critical in making an accurate and timely diagnosis.
- Many times, complaint of ankle pain is when a patient may first seek treatments for flexible flatfoot deformity.

INTRODUCTION

Adult acquired flatfoot deformity is generally associated with a collapsing medial longitudinal arch and progressive loss of strength of the tibialis posterior tendon. It is most commonly associated with posterior tibial tendon (PTT) dysfunction (PTTD) that can have an arthritic or traumatic cause. With an increasing population of obese patients, the often misdiagnosed and overlooked PTTD will only continue to present more often in the foot and ankle specialist's office. This article focuses on the anatomy, classification, and pathomechanics of the flexible adult flatfoot.

CLASSIFICATION
Johnson and Strom

Many classification systems have been described in the literature formulated from clinical findings, radiographic findings, and/or etiology of the pathology. In 1989, Johnson and Strom[1] introduced a classification system that was intended to correlate the presentation, physical findings, and radiographic findings that would ultimately guide surgical intervention and still remains the most widely used.

Stage 1, tenosynovitis is predominant. There is an absence of hindfoot valgus, too many toes, and patients are generally able to perform a single heel raise. Tendon

Relationship Disclosure: The authors have no disclosures to report.
West Houston Medical and Surgical Residency Program PMSR/RRA, West Houston Medical Center, 12121 Richmond Avenue, Suite 417, Houston, TX 77082, USA
* Corresponding author.
E-mail address: JeremyLWalters@gmail.com

length is preserved and patients elicit pain with direct palpation of the tendon distal to the medial malleolus.

Stage 2 is typically when the first sign of deformity presents. The tendon has developed degeneration and elongation and a hindfoot valgus is appreciated with possible forefoot abduction (**Fig. 1**). Patients may be able to perform a single heel raise in this stage but as the dysfunction progresses the ability is lost (**Fig. 2**). It is important to remember that in this stage, the deformity remains flexible. A trend in recent years has been to subdivide this category into "A" and "B," where the "A" group represents patients with medial pain and the ability to perform a single heel raise. "B" group patients have fibular impingement pain and incompetence of the PTT.

Stage 3 is for the patient that has developed a rigid deformity. The examiner is unable to correct the forefoot abduction or hindfoot valgus on examination, patients typically complain of only lateral pain, and patients are unable to perform single heel raise.

Stage 4 is reserved for the patient that progresses to ankle joint involvement. The dysfunction leads to a valgus talus and eventually attenuation of the deltoid ligament. The once subfibular impingement pain is now pain generally related to ankle arthritis.

ANATOMY

Pertinent anatomy of the flexible flatfoot deformity involves more than simply a failure of the PTT. The calcaneonavicular ligament, deltoid complex, and the articular involvement of the talonavicular joint (TNJ) should always be taken into consideration when evaluating any flatfoot deformity.

PTT

The PTT has origins on the posterior aspect of the tibia, fibula, and interosseous membrane. It was Morimoto[2] in 1983 that suggested the fibular origin is the strongest and evolutionarily newer than the tibial side. It is the more lateral origin of the muscle that improves the lever arm and provides greater inversion of the foot. The tendon crosses the medial aspect of the posterior talus, the medial aspect of the talar neck, and the inferior surface of the inferocalcaneonavicular ligament and is located above the sustentaculum tali.[3] According to Bloome and colleagues,[4] just in front of the navicular tuberosity the PTT splits into three bands: (1) anterior, (2) middle, and (3) posterior. The anterior band is the largest and a direct continuation of the tendon that inserts into the navicular tuberosity, the inferior surface of the navicular-cuneiform joint, and the plantar aspect of the first metatarsal cuneiform joint. The middle component

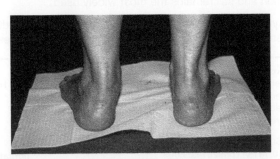

Fig. 1. Development of hindfoot valgus is noted.

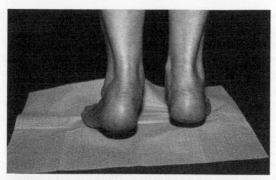

Fig. 2. The right heel goes into varus while the left hindfoot remains in valgus.

is a very deep band that continues distally into the sole of the foot and inserts into the cuneiforms and cuboid. The posterior component originates before tendon insertion on the tuberosity and courses laterally, inserting onto the anterior aspect of the sustentaculum tali. The width of the tendinous bands as a percentage of the whole is anterior 65%, middle band 15%, and posterior band 20%.[3,4] The importance of this tendon cannot be overlooked; Jahss[5] noted the normal inversion strength of the calf muscles to be 12 to 15 pounds of torque. With a rupture of the PTT, the torque of the calf muscles decreases to 3 to 6 pounds of torque.

The vascular supply to the PTT remains a controversial topic. The posterior tibial artery is the primary blood supply to the tendon, although Sarrafian[3] reports the insertion might receive its blood supply from branches off the dorsalis pedis artery. In 28 cadaveric specimens, Frey and colleagues[6] identified a hypovascular zone 40 mm proximal to the PTT insertion that begins at the level of the medial malleolus and, interestingly, there was no mesotenon present at this level. In the study control, the flexor digitorum longus tendon, no such zone existed and a consistent vascularity was noted. Peterson and colleagues[7] attempted to replicate the study using a different technique and found an avascular zone rather than a hypovascular zone at the level of the medial malleolus. A third theory proposed by Mosier and colleagues[8] stated the PTT actually contained neovasculization of the tendon in the degenerative region caused by the increase in mucin and myxoid degeneration and attributed the degeneration to a collagen disorder in place of a vascular cause of the PTT degeneration.

Plantar Calcaneonavicular Ligament

First known as the ligamentum neglectum and as part of the tibiocalcaneonavicular ligament, the plantar calcaneonavicular ligament was later determined by Lane[9] to be a separate ligament. The plantar calcaneonavicular is typically described as consisting of two bundles, superomedial and inferior. Many anatomic descriptions exist in the literature; Sarrafian and colleagues[3] and Davis and colleagues[10] have each offered their own descriptions but it has generally been accepted that the superomedial bundle is subject to stress at the level of the TNJ and as a result is covered dorsally by fibrocartilage, thus making it the strongest and broadest of the two bundles that form the acetabulum pedis.[11] The superomedial bundle is triangular and shaped like a hammock. The ligament originates from the middle facet and sustentaculum tali of the subtalar joint and inserts onto the navicular tuberosity and the superior aspect of the medial side of the navicular articular margin. The inferoplantar bundle is a short and broad ligament. The origin is classically described as between the anterior and middle articular facets of the subtalar joint and inserting into navicular beak laterally.

Histologically, there appears to be an absence of elastic fibers within the complex,[12,13] thus possibly making reference to the plantar calcaneonavicular ligament as the spring ligament to be inaccurate because no elastic properties exist within it. The dorsal and central third of the superomedial bundle is avascular with the calcaneal branches of the medial plantar artery supplying the proximal aspect of the ligament and the distal third receiving its vascular supply from the navicular branches of the medial plantar artery.[10] The ligament complex serves as static support for the head of the talus, provides support to the TNJ, and provides medial longitudinal arch support.[14]

Deltoid Ligament Complex

The deltoid ligament complex is a delta-shaped, relatively strong and broad complex that functions to connect the leg and the foot. There are many different descriptions of the anatomy of the complex but most authors agree that the deltoid ligament is composed of two layers (superficial and deep) separated by a fat pad and each layer has several components. One of the most common descriptions of the deltoid ligament is by Milner and Soames,[15] which is briefly reviewed next.

The superficial layer is composed of the tibionavicular ligament (TNL), superficial posterior talotibial ligament, and the calcaneotibial ligament. The TNL extends from the anterior inferior aspect of the medial malleolus to the navicular tuberosity where it blends with the calcaneonavicular ligament in the foot and has been noted to be the weakest component of the deltoid complex. The superficial posterior talotibial ligament runs from the posterior inferior aspect of the medial malleolus to the medial tubercle of the posterior talar process and often blends with deep fibers and functions to prevent posterior displacement of the talus and excessive ankle dorsiflexion. Extending from the medial malleolar colliculi to the medial surface of the sustentaculum tali and lying deep to the flexor digitorum longus tendon is the calcaneotibial ligament, which functions to limit eversion.

The deep layer consists of the anterior talotibial ligament and the deep posterior talotibial ligament. The anterior talotibial ligament extends from the anterior colliculus of the medial malleolus to the medial aspect of the talar neck and is often intertwined with fibers of the TNL. The deep posterior talotibial ligament runs from the posterior colliculus of the medial malleolus to the medial tubercle of the posterior process of the talus.

The deltoid complex serves many purposes but overall serves to provide stability to the ankle joint, act as a primary medial ankle stabilizer, and prevents valgus tilting of the talus.

TNJ

The ovoid, convex talar head articulates with the concavity of the navicular and the surrounding ligamentous structures. Static ligamentous support and the dynamic support from the tibialis posterior and foot flexors are important in allowing normal talar head motion and function of the transverse tarsal joint.

The navicular receives blood supply from several sources. The dorsal aspect arises from a branch of the dorsalis pedis and the plantar aspect from the medial plantar artery. The tuberosity has a network formed from the dorsalis pedis and the medial plantar artery, thus giving the bone a rich vascularization network. The blood supply to the talus is well documented.[16–18]

PATHOMECHANICS

The stabilization of the medial arch by the PTT involves static and dynamic vectors. Static support theories generally fall into two categories: those who believe the foot is a truss and those who believe it acts as a beam. The truss theory is supported by Lapidus's work,[19] who stated that a truss works by creating two planks or struts that meet at an apex with base support by a tie rod, creating a triangle. Translating this to the foot, the tie rod is the plantar fascia and the tarsal bones the struts. As the apex is loaded, the forces are applied to the planks and tensile forces to the tie rod. As long as the plantar fascia remains intact, the truss holds firm. This theory was also supported by Hicks,[20] who is most noted for his support of the plantar fascia and the windlass mechanism. This concept is important to remember when having patients perform a single heel rise to test the integrity of the PTT. Patients with an incompetent PTT are unable to perform a single heel rise. However, often patients are able to cheat by recruiting other muscles or by raising up on both tip toes and then balancing on one foot. It is quite plausible that a patient would be unable to perform a single heel raise because of PTT insufficiency but be able to maintain a heel rise once up because of the plantar fascia plantarflexing the metatarsal heads, thus leading to inversion of the heel. Patients have essentially bypassed the PTT mechanism to accomplish the task.

Sarrafian[3] proposed the beam theory, which is based on a less rigid construct. He believed the foot acted as a beam that sags when loaded. Compression forces exist on the convex side and tensile forces on the concave side. The curved component of the beam consists of midfoot bones, leading tensile forces to affect the concave side or the plantar foot ligaments and the calcaneonavicular ligament.

Dynamic support is based on the role of the tibialis posterior muscle and intrinsic foot muscles. Tension along the tibialis posterior adducts and plantar flexes the navicular on the talar head. This enables the tendon to prevent the longitudinal arch from collapse. With the calcaneocuboid ligament, the cuboid is able to exert a medial pull on the calcaneus, thus providing additional support to the talar head through the anterior and middle facets. The tibialis posterior muscle, a stance phase muscle, produces inversion of the hindfoot and acts to oppose the peroneus brevis. During mid-stance, the posterior tibial muscle contraction causes subtalar inversion, locking the transverse tarsal joints resulting in a rigid lever for propulsion.[21,22]

With PTTD, the balance is altered and shifted toward the peroneals with greater hindfoot eversion and ligamentous tension during stance. The gastrocnemius-soleus then acts at the TNJ creating excessive midfoot stress, which leads to midfoot abduction and early heel lift. It is important to remember that with the hindfoot in valgus, the triceps surae becomes a powerful pronator instead of supinator of the foot during heel rise. The equinus force is only increased with extension of the knee during heel rise, which can ultimately increase the force of the Achilles by 30%.[23] It is this repetitive biomechanical alteration of gait that results in the progressive midfoot collapse, forefoot abduction (relative lengthening of the medial column), and excessive hindfoot valgus (relative shortening of the lateral column).[22]

The exact structures that attenuate and the subsequent structural foot changes remain an area of debate. Hansen[24] and Van Boerum and Sangeorzan[25] agreed with Brodsky's description previously described and termed this peritalar subluxation. They believe it is the movement of the talus that causes retrograde eversion of the calcaneus leading to the progression of the deformity. Deland and colleagues[26] were able to demonstrate the importance of the medial soft tissue failure in cadaver models by sectioning the calcaneonavicular complex and posterior medial structures. The loss of static ligamentous support of the arch has been identified to be one of the most critical steps in collapse of the medial longitudinal arch, of which Deland and colleagues[27,28] demonstrates the failure of the plantar calcaneonavicular ligament to be the most instrumental.

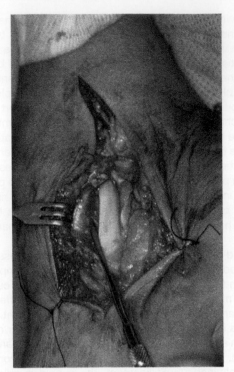

Fig. 3. Pannus formation within tendon sheath of tibialis posterior tendon.

A flexible adult acquired flatfoot deformity is most commonly associated with PTTD. The biomechanical overloading as described can lead to chronic microtrauma, which the tendon is unable to adapt to with advancing age, creating the pathologic cycle weakening the static stabilizers of the foot.

Chronic inflammation of the tibialis posterior tendon has also been associated with inflammatory joint diseases, such as rheumatoid arthritis, systemic lupus erythymatosis, and seronegative arthropathies.[29–32] Michelson and colleagues[33] found that 64% of patients with rheumatoid arthritis have some form of PTTD (**Fig. 3**). When patients present with chronic tenosynovitis that fails to respond to medical management or intraoperative findings are suggestive of inflammatory disease, the appropriate clinical and serologic testing should be completed.

SUMMARY

The adult acquired flat foot is a complex, multifaceted pathology that requires the foot and ankle specialist to have a full understanding of the anatomy involved and the biomechanics to be able to accurately perform a physical examination, make a diagnosis, and plan less aggressive surgical intervention if needed. Left untreated or undiagnosed, the peritalar subluxation may progress to dislocation and severe degenerative joint disease.

REFERENCES

1. Johnson KA, Strom DE. Tibialis posterior tendon dysfunction. Clin Orthop Relat Res 1989;(239):L196–206.

2. Morimoto I. Notes on architecture of tibialis posterior muscle in man. Kaibogaku Zasshi 1983;58:74–80.
3. Sarrafian S. Anatomy of the foot and ankle: descriptive, topographical. 3rd edition. Philadelphia: JB Lippincott; 2011.
4. Bloome DM, Marymont JV, Varner KE. Variations on the insertion of the posterior tibialis tendon: a cadaveric study. Foot Ankle Int 2003;24(10):780–3.
5. Jahss MH. Spontaneous rupture of the tibialis posterior tendon: clinical findings, tenographic studies and a new technique of repair. Foot Ankle 1982;3: 158–66.
6. Frey C, Shereff M, Greenidge N. Vascularity of the posterior tibial tendon. J Bone Joint Surg Am 1990;72:884–8.
7. Peterson W, Hohmann G, Stein V, et al. The blood supply of the posterior tibial tendon. J Bone Joint Surg Br 2002;84:141–4.
8. Mosier SM, Lucas DR, Pomeroy G, et al. Pathology of the posterior tibial tendon in posterior tibial tendon insufficiency. Foot Ankle Int 1998;19:520–4.
9. Lane AS. The causation, pathology and physiology of several of the deformities which develop during young life. Guys Hosp Rep 1887;44:254.
10. Davis WH, Sobel M, Dicarlo EF, et al. Gross, histological, and microvascular anatomy and biomechanical testing of the spring ligament complex. Foot Ankle Int 1996;17:95–102.
11. Patil V, Ebraheim N, Frogrameni A, et al. Morphometric dimensions of the calcaneonavicular (spring) ligament. Foot Ankle Int 2007;28(8):927–32.
12. Hardy RH. Observations on the structure and properties of the plantar calcaneonavicular ligament in man. J Anat 1951;85:135–9.
13. Burgos J, Loncharich E, Macklin Vadell A, et al. Vascularización del ligamento calcáneo-escafoideo. Tobillo y Pie/Tornazelo e Pé 2010;2(2):28–33.
14. Rule J, Yao L, Seeger LL. Spring ligament of the ankle: normal MR anatomy. Am J Roentgenol 1993;161:1241–4.
15. Milner CE, Soames RW. Anatomy of the collateral ligaments of the human ankle joint. Foot Ankle 1998;19:757–60.
16. Haliburton R, Sullivan A, Kelly P, et al. The extra-osseous and intra-osseous blood supply of the talus. J Bone Joint Surg Am 1958;40:1115–20.
17. Summers NJ, Murdoch MM. Fractures of the talus: a comprehensive review. Clin Podiatr Med Surg 2012;29(2):187–203.
18. Prasarn ML, Miller AN, Dyke JP, et al. Arterial anatomy of the talus: a cadaver and gadolinium-enhanced MRI study. Foot Ankle Int 2010;31(11):987–93.
19. Lapidus PW. Kinesiology and mechanical anatomy of the tarsal joints. Clin Orthop Relat Res 1963;30:20–36.
20. Hicks JH. The mechanics of the foot. II: the plantar aponeurosis and the arch. J Anat 1954;88:25–30.
21. Mann RA, Coughlin MJ. Surgery of the foot and ankle. 6th edition. St Louis (MO): Mosby Inc; 1993.
22. Brodsky JW. Preliminary gait analysis results after posterior tibial tendon reconstruction: a prospective study. Foot Ankle Int 2004;25(2):96–100.
23. Mann RA. Biomechanics of the foot. Atlas of orthotics: biomechanical principles and application. St Louis (MO): C.V. Mosby; 1975. p. 264.
24. Hansen ST. Progressive symptomatic flat foot (lateral peritalar subluxation). In: Hansen ST, editor. Functional reconstruction of the foot and ankle. Philadelphia: Lippincott Williams & Wilkins; 2000. p. 195–207.
25. Van Boerum DH, Sangeorzan BJ. Biomechanics and pathophysiology of flat foot. Foot Ankle Clin 2003;8:419–30.

26. Deland JT, Arnoczky SP, Thompson FM. Adult acquired flatfoot deformity at the talonavicular joint: reconstruction of the spring ligament in an in vitro model. Foot Ankle 1992;13(6):327–32.
27. Deland JT, de Asia RJ, Sung IH, et al. Posterior tibial tendon insufficiency: which ligaments are involved? Foot Ankle Int 2005;26:427–35.
28. Deland JT. The adult-acquired flatfoot and spring ligament complex. Pathology and implications for treatment. Foot Ankle Clin 2001;6:129–35.
29. Crunkshank B. Lesions of joints and tendon sheaths in systematic lupus erythematosus. Ann Rheum Dis 1959;18:111–9.
30. Downey DJ, Simpkin PA, Mack LA, et al. Tibialis posterior tendon rupture: a cause of the rheumatoid flatfoot. Arthritis Rheum 1988;31:441–6.
31. Michelson J, Easley M, Wigley FM, et al. Posterior tibial tendon dysfunction in rheumatoid arthritis. Foot Ankle Int 1995;16:156–61.
32. Myerson M, Soloman G, Shereff M. Posterior tibial dysfunction: its association with seronegative inflammatory disease. Foot Ankle Int 1989;9:215–9.
33. Michelson J, Easley M, Wigley FM, et al. Foot and ankle problems in rheumatoid arthritis. Foot Ankle Int 1994;15:608–13.

Nonoperative Management of Adult Flatfoot Deformities

Roger Marzano, CPO, Cped

KEYWORDS

- Flatfoot deformities • Footwear • Footwear modifications • Foot orthoses
- Ankle foot orthoses • Short articulating AFO

KEY POINTS

- There are many conservative options available to the patient with a flatfoot disorder, from simple shoe modifications to patellar tendon bearing ankle foot orthoses.
- There is increasingly more clinical evidence to support the efficacy of conservatively managing this pathologic abnormality.
- As surgical techniques are analyzed and improved, so too are the footwear, foot orthoses, and ankle foot orthoses.

INTRODUCTION

Managing those with adult flatfoot deformities can be quite challenging, and the methods and devices used are wide-ranging based on the experience of the managing physician and the experience of the provider of the orthotic devices. A thorough biomechanical assessment is paramount to provide the most successful treatment due to the wide range of pathologic abnormalities and pathomechanics that lead to this painful disorder.

Specific Diagnosis

A well-defined diagnosis with specific classification of the deformity is necessary for successful management of those with adult flatfoot deformities. The reasoning behind specificity in diagnoses is to allow the orthotist or pedorthist to determine if the structure of the foot can be corrected and to what degree. For example, the ability to influence the alignment of the foot and ankle would vary from correction to accommodation if the patient had tarsal coalition versus stage II posterior tibial tendon dysfunction (PTTD). The patient that presents with a rigid coalition would not respond to aggressive correction in the build of the orthosis, whereas a patient with stage II

Yanke Bionics Clinics, Inc, 303 West Exchange Street, Akron, OH 44302, USA
E-mail address: rmarzano@yankebionics.com

Clin Podiatr Med Surg 31 (2014) 337–347
http://dx.doi.org/10.1016/j.cpm.2014.03.007
0891-8422/14/$ – see front matter © 2014 Elsevier Inc. All rights reserved.

PTTD could, and should, have some correction of the alignment in the orthosis of choice. That is just one example of why specificity of the diagnosis, which led to the resultant flatfoot deformity, is so important. The more information that the prescribing physician can provide to the orthotist or pedorthist, the more accurately one can then provide the proper correction in alignment during the impression process for orthoses. Diagnostic specificity also determines the rigidity of material selection when formulating the construction of the orthosis; therefore, any direction as to the mechanical objectives as the prescribing physician sees fit will enhance the outcomes of conservative management. Insurance requirements today also depend on specific diagnostic information, as well as defined mechanical objectives of orthotic management to determine coverage for services. Good prescribing physician documentation is key to assisting patients in obtaining coverage for orthotic services.

PATHOMECHANICS AND BIOMECHANICAL ASSESSMENT

A successful outcome with this patient population directly correlates to proper patient and biomechanical assessment. Patient assessment should include any previous foot surgeries, the prior use of orthoses and other devices tried, any previous injuries contributing to their diagnosis, and any other medical conditions that may contribute to their condition as presented.

The most common alignment deficiencies seen in those with adult flatfoot deformity are forefoot varus, hypermobility of the first ray, and a congenitally or iatrogenically shortened first ray, which often presents with transfer metatarsalgia. Other alignment deviations commonly seen in this patient population are excessive calcaneal valgus with resultant subfibular impingement, peritalar subluxation, and equinus contractures noted in most (**Fig. 1**). In late stage II and stage III tibialis posterior tendon dysfunction patients, one may see stress fractures of the distal fibula and lateral column symptoms due to the compressive forces to the lateral articular structures of the hindfoot. Other concomitant pathologic abnormalities commonly managed with these patients are hallux limitus or rigidus, tibialis posterior tendinosis or rupture, tarsal coalition, accessory navicular, midfoot osteoarthrosis, Charcot osteoarthropathy, and even some failed or nonunions of single, double, or triple arthrodeses. Patients who have had previous ankle arthrodeses or malaligned arthrodeses will often, over time, develop a secondary flatfoot deformity due to the subtalar and midtarsal articulations becoming mobile in dorsiflexion to compensate for the loss of talocrural mobility created by the ankle fusion.

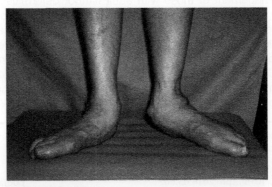

Fig. 1. Adult with flatfoot deformity.

With a good diagnosis in hand, a standard biomechanical assessment can then be performed, which should include evaluation of the forefoot to hindfoot relationship to determine the degree of forefoot varus that may be contributing to their presentation of hindfoot valgus. Other important factors to determine in the biomechanical examination are the amount of calcaneal inversion or eversion to determine if the alignment is flexible or fixed, such as those with a coalition or previous fusion. The examination of hindfoot mobility will designate either correction or accommodation of the hindfoot alignment with the orthotic intervention. Another critical assessment is to determine the presence and degree of gastroc-soleus contractures. Anyone caring for this group of patients will see that the ankle contractures cause the midtarsal joints to compensate for lost ankle range of motion. The patients with contractures must have allowances for compensatory subtalar and midtarsal collapse built into their orthotic device. These patients are prone to be overcorrected when making the model for an orthosis and subsequently put the device in their closet instead of in their shoe. It is paramount to recognize that these individuals have not seen subtalar neutral for several years and will not tolerate overcorrection of the compensatory alignment deviations that occur in later stages of those with adult flatfoot disorders. One rule of thumb that has been beneficial to think of is that the more flexible the foot structure is, the more rigid the device can be, and, conversely, the more rigid the foot structure, the more accommodative the device should be. Proper and detailed diagnoses, combined with a thorough patient and biomechanical assessment, will enhance any lower extremity practitioner's outcomes and, more importantly, provide pain relief and nonoperative options for this group.

NONOPERATIVE MANAGEMENT OPTIONS

There are more treatment options today for those with a flatfoot disorder than ever before. Tools for managing those with flatfoot disorders often include a combination of footwear changes, footwear modifications, custom foot orthoses, and custom ankle foot orthoses (AFO). It may be necessary to use one or more of these conservative tools for successful management of flatfeet. Recognizing the importance of the role of footwear for this patient group is the best starting point to discussing management options with your patient.

FOOTWEAR CONSIDERATIONS FOR FLATFEET

Footwear alone can make a tremendous impact on better foot function and alignment, and many patients present with shoes that are inadequate to provide good support. A frank discussion with your patient about footwear is a good starting point to explain construction and characteristics in shoes that would be beneficial to them. With today's Internet purchases of footwear increasing, it is important to recommend the flatfoot patient to have their foot measured for adequate sizing and fit. One common misconception that is often overused is to have them purchase a "running shoe," which is often constructed using a curved last (model in which a shoe is constructed over) designed to supinate the foot. Therefore, essentially, it is an adducted shoe on a group of patients that present with significant forefoot abduction, which leads to painful corns and callusing to the lesser toes because of the abduction of the forefoot and crowding of the lesser toes in an adducted shoe shape. The narrow midfoot in running shoes also allows for the pronated midfoot to overpower the upper and get minimal midfoot support where they need it the most. With that in mind, it is better to recommend a "walking shoe" or a shoe constructed specifically for walking, which will normally have a leather, versus a fabric, upper that increases wear life of the shoe and better "molds" to the shape of the foot as the shoe breaks in. Walking shoes normally have a wider midfoot region for better arch support and, depending on the manufacturer and model types, will have multiple widths available for better fitting and for accommodating orthotic devices.

A cross-training design athletic shoe is another type of footwear construction that works well to support the flatfoot structure, is designed for lateral motion activities, and serves to provide better hindfoot control, which is optimum for this patient group.

Other valuable construction characteristics that can be suggested are to have a lace up or Velcro closure, versus a slip-on-type shoe, to adjust for the use of an orthotic device. A firm heel counter will help resist calcaneal valgus and should be found in most better-quality walking and supportive footwear.

There is a small group of patients with significant deformities who cannot be fit in commercially available athletic or comfort footwear and who will need to be fit with custom-made shoes. Particularly, custom shoes may be better suited for the flatfoot patient with compromised sensation secondary to diabetic or peripheral neuropathy. Any patient who has failed quality, professionally fit footwear, will best be served in custom-made shoes.

There is greater availability of stylish yet supportive shoes to recommend to your patient, and it is wise for the managing physician to be conversant in footwear characteristics to secure a better outcome with any conservative intervention. Every person you treat for a flatfoot disorder should have their feet measured every time they purchase a new pair of shoes because of the progressive nature of this disorder. People tend to equate the quality of the shoe with the price that they paid, which is not necessarily true because an expensive poorly fit shoe can be just as detrimental as an inexpensive one. Successful management of flatfoot disorders should begin with appropriately fit and constructed footwear, which best matches the patient's size, activity level, occupational demands, and severity of their deformity.

COMMON FOOTWEAR MODIFICATIONS

There are several common modifications to footwear that can enhance the function and support the patient derives from the footwear and modifications alone. The medial counter reinforcement to the shoe supports the medial column of the foot by widening the base of support under the longitudinal arch and prevents the medial collapse of the shoe over time (**Fig. 2**). This modification serves those who have some degree of correction available in the earlier stages of posterior tibialis tendon dysfunction. For those who have fixed, collapsed hindfoot and midfoot deformities, performing a split and widen modification to the shoe serves to widen the midfoot of the shoe internally and accommodates the significant medial prominences seen in the later stages of this

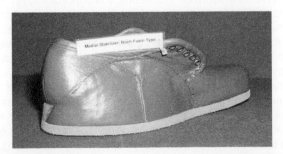

Fig. 2. Medial counter reinforcement.

disorder (**Fig. 3**). This modification may be tried before prescribing more expensive and less-appealing custom footwear.

In more involved feet with significant plantar deformities, it may be necessary to excavate the midsole of the shoe under the plantar prominence to offload a preulcerative callus further (**Fig. 4**). This excavation of the midsole of the shoe can be useful in the forefoot as well for a transfer lesion under the second metatarsal, seen in those with significant acquired forefoot varus. This modification, coined the "drill and fill," is useful anytime a plantar prominence needs off-loaded anywhere within the shoe.

Rocker soles have been useful in caring for rigid flatfoot deformities to facilitate normal heel to toe gait while minimizing bending stresses, which can be beneficial to alleviate osteoarthritic symptoms. The rocker sole can benefit those with ankle or subtalar arthrodeses by reducing compensatory painful range of motion of the tarsal-metatarsal joints or the metatarsal phalangeal articulations.

Footwear modifications can elevate clinical outcomes, but are not always followed through with because of lack of coverage by most insurers for shoe modifications and the frequency in which they have to be done with multiple shoe changes. If done correctly, the benefits of shoe modifications will outweigh the cost and may prevent or delay surgical intervention.

CUSTOM FOOT ORTHOSES

Custom foot orthoses are commonly prescribed in the early stages of adult flatfoot disorders and have volumes of research to support their efficacy of use. There are a wide variety of construction types and material compositions being used. The concept of the more flexible the foot structure, the more rigid the orthosis should be, and the more rigid the foot structure, the softer, more accommodative the orthosis should be, has served this author well when providing orthoses in clinical practice. Regardless of the construction design or material composition used in the orthotic fabrications, sound biomechanical principles musts be followed in supporting these foot structures. Subtalar neutral has been the gold standard when taking impressions for foot orthoses, but this group of patients will not respond favorably if overcorrected in their casting. This group's non-weight-bearing resting alignment is most often their "neutral" position. The clinical presentation for most of these patients includes acquired forefoot varus, hypermobility of the first ray, forefoot abduction, a declined

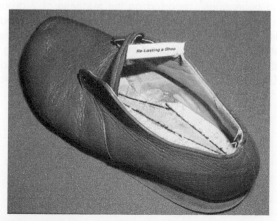

Fig. 3. Split and widen midsole.

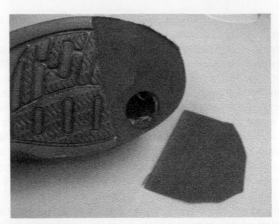

Fig. 4. Drill and fill modification.

talocalcaneal angle, and greater resting valgus of the hindfoot. Also the effect of equinus contractures seen concurrently with the adult flatfoot must be taken into consideration. If the orthosis takes away all, or too much, of their compensatory midfoot accommodation, then the orthosis will feel like a rock in their shoe and will not be worn successfully, because the midtarsal collapse compensated for the lost talocrural motion. It is as much an art as it is a science when determining the best position to mold the foot to provide a comfortable, yet functional, orthosis. A medially posted orthosis, with both hindfoot and forefoot posting, has been effective to reduce hindfoot valgus and bring the ground up to the first ray for those with forefoot varus or first ray hypermobility (**Fig. 5**). If the patient has a significant equinus contracture, a heel lift may need to be incorporated as well. The use of a heel lift can also reduce the sensation of too much arch, which a patient may experience if slightly overcorrected in the casting process, and can be helpful if the medial hindfoot posting alone was not sufficient to reduce subfibular impingement symptoms.

When a patient progresses to the point that their foot orthoses are no longer effective to control their symptoms, then a University of California Berkeley Laboratory (UCBL) orthosis may be the next to try before going to an AFO (**Fig. 6**). The UCBL is a rigid foot orthosis designed to control the triplanar motion of the hindfoot and midfoot. Chao and colleagues[1] reported on the success of 2 groups, one treated with a UCBL and one treated with a molded ankle foot orthosis; good to excellent results were demonstrated with a UCBL. One's clinical success with the UCBL is due in part to 2 qualifications—the experience of the practitioner providing the device, and the proper patient selection for fitting. Patients best served and most successful in the use of a UCBL are those with flexible, or easily correctable, midfoot and hindfoot

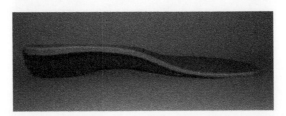

Fig. 5. Medially posted foot orthosis.

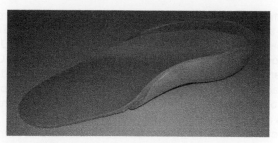

Fig. 6. UCBL orthosis.

alignment, and those with late stage I or stage II tibialis posterior tendon dysfunction, as classified by Johnson and Strom.[2] Imhauser and colleagues[3] reported that the UCBL significantly restored all the parameters of the arch, including the calcaneal angle, inclination of the first metatarsal, with increased talar, navicular, and arch heights. A UCBL has been frequently prescribed for those with tarsal coalitions, but a soft interface may need to be incorporated to increase patient compliance and comfort in this group of patients because of the rigidity of their foot structures.

There are several factors that insure successful orthotic intervention with custom foot orthoses, including the skill of the practitioner in assessing the pathomechanics as presented, a specific diagnosis with mechanical objectives, and the proper posting of the orthosis, as indicated by the biomechanical examination. When these 3 tools are optimized, the patient has a pain-relieving outcome.

ANKLE FOOT ORTHOSES FOR FLATFOOT DEFORMITIES

It is prudent to first try over-the-counter or noncustom AFO so in the event of continued symptoms, there will be documentation to support the need of a custom-made AFO. Medicare and many insurers are closely analyzing AFO claims for documentation to support the need of a custom AFO versus an off-the-shelf design. In the early stages of this disorder, and in the absence of deformity, an off-the-shelf sports-type supramalleolar ankle brace may be beneficial to the appropriate patient. When and if that treatment fails, a custom AFO will be indicated.

It has been well documented that the use of AFO for the treatment of flatfoot disorders is successful particularly for those with tibialis posterior tendon dysfunction.[1,4,5] The studies varied slightly, but improvement of symptoms was reported in 50% to 90% of those studied with good compliance. The most common types of AFO prescribed are the Richey, Arizona, or a short articulating AFO design (SAAFO).

The Arizona AFO has been widely used for the treatment of flatfoot disorders and works to reduce midfoot, hindfoot, and talocrural motion. Good clinical research is available to substantiate the outcomes.

Another popular and well-documented AFO for the treatment of flatfoot disorders is the Richie AFO. This design has 2 independent struts harnessed together by circumferential strapping with a functional foot orthotic footplate that the hinges and uprights are attached to. This orthosis has been researched and proven to be a great treatment tool for those in the early stages of a flatfoot disorder.

A lesser documented, but highly effective, AFO that has gained credibility and increased use among podiatric and orthopedic physicians, developed by this author, is the SAAFO. The SAAFO uses a thermoplastic anterior shell to bridge the medial and lateral segments anteriorly and serves to harness and reduce the internal tibial rotation associated with midtarsal and hindfoot collapse, simulating the control of a hinged ski boot (**Fig. 7**). The short anterior shell eases application and allows the device to remain in the shoe and be applied with the shoe, versus first donning the AFO, and then struggling with the shoe application. Another unique feature of the SAAFO is the incorporation of a full-length soft foot orthosis into the footplate for medial hindfoot and forefoot posting and to cushion any plantar bony prominences or provide an aperture for a depressed or prominent metatarsal head. This device is essentially an external triple arthrodesis and has had good patient acceptance.[6]

In later stages of the flatfoot disorder when there is the need for more extensive control of range of motion, the next type of AFO commonly prescribed is a solid ankle AFO (**Fig. 8**). This AFO is indicated for those with associated degenerative arthrosis of the ankle, those with significant subfibular impingement, or those whose symptoms are no longer alleviated with an articulated AFO. Again, a soft interface should be incorporated to aid in impact absorption and posting objectives, and to enhance patient compliance. This orthosis can be composed of different densities or rigidities of plastic to grade the amount of restriction of mobility required to control the patient's symptoms. The use of a rocker-soled shoe modification is helpful for patients wearing a solid ankle AFO to facilitate a smoother, more energy-efficient gait when immobilizing the talocrural and hindfoot articulations.

In those patients with end-stage flatfoot deformities or nonoperative patients, it may be necessary to axially unload the ankle and hindfoot with the use of a patellar tendon–bearing AFO (PTB) AFO (**Fig. 9**). This orthosis is useful for those with a flatfoot deformity that may have diabetic or peripheral neuropathy, with increased chances of developing Charcot osteoarthropathy. This device offloads the ankle and hindfoot by loading the proximal calf anatomy and using hydrostatic compression of the soft tissue of the calf. This device can be fabricated from thermoplastics or a metal and molding leather calf lacer, for those with fluctuating edema secondary to lymphedema or venous stasis, or for those that are larger in size. The PTB or calf lacer is normally the last orthotic alternative when managing those with adult acquired flatfoot deformities (**Fig. 10**).

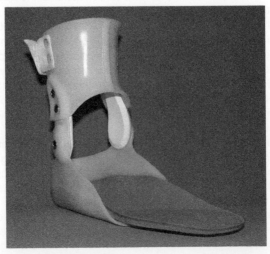

Fig. 7. Short articulating AFO, or SAAFO.

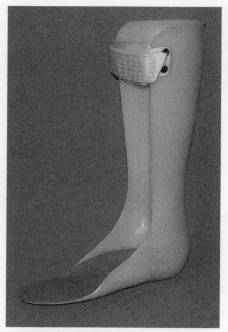

Fig. 8. Solid ankle AFO.

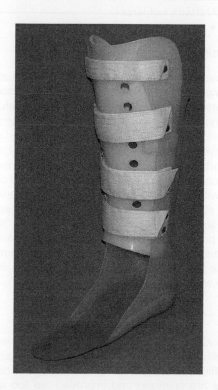

Fig. 9. PTB AFO.

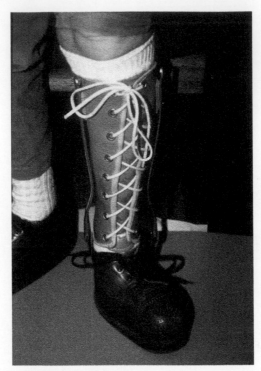

Fig. 10. Double upright AFO with calf lacer.

POSTOPERATIVE CONSIDERATIONS

The postoperative management of any flatfoot disorder usually involves providing support to the remaining architecture and providing more accommodative devices; this is because the surgeries to correct the foot deformity often involve tendon transfers and/or bony realignment, and, in some cases, fusions combined with soft tissue and osteotomies to provide better residual alignment. The most common devices provided to those who have had reconstructive flatfoot surgery are quality supportive footwear, custom foot orthoses, and, in some more involved cases, the use of an ankle foot orthosis. It is the goal of the surgeon to eliminate the need of an AFO, but in some severe cases or those with postoperative complications, nonunions, or residual malalignment, the AFO may still be needed during the healing process. The most common postoperative complications include nonunions, forefoot to hindfoot malalignment created by a hindfoot procedure without adequately correcting the associated acquired forefoot varus, and lateral column pain secondary to a residual varus hindfoot alignment. All the same pedorthic and orthotic devices discussed earlier would be useful in treating those with postoperative alignment issues.

SUMMARY

There are many conservative options available to the patient with a flatfoot disorder, from simple shoe modifications to PTB AFO. There is increasingly more clinical evidence to support the efficacy of conservatively managing this pathologic abnormality. As surgical techniques are analyzed and improved, so too are the footwear, foot orthoses, and AFO. The foot care team should include the pedorthist and orthotist to succeed in managing those with this challenging pathologic abnormality. Taking away pain while improving function for any patient is one of the most rewarding aspects of clinical foot care, and the information covered in this article should arm the practitioner, or surgeon, with viable alternatives to surgical management.

REFERENCES

1. Chao W, Wapner KL, Lee TH, et al. Non-operative management of posterior tibial tendon dysfunction. Foot Ankle Int 1996;17(12):736–41.
2. Johnson KA, Strom DE. Tibialis posterior tendon dysfunction. Clin Orthop 1989; 239:196–206.
3. Imhauser CW, Abidi NA, Frankel DZ, et al. Biomechanical evaluation of the efficacy of external shoe stabilizers in the conservative treatment acquired flat foot deformity. Foot Ankle Int 2002;23(8):727–37.
4. Augustyn JF, Lin SS, Berberian WS, et al. Non operative treatment of adult acquired flat foot with the Arizona brace. Foot Ankle Clin 2003;8(3):491–502.
5. Myerson MS. Adult acquired flat foot deformity: treatment of dysfunction of the posterior tibial tendon. J Bone Joint Surg Am 1966;78:780–92.
6. Marzano R. The shorter cure for tibialis posterior tendon dysfunction. Biomechanics 1995;2:57–61.

Flexible Adult Flatfoot

Soft Tissue Procedures

Jeremy L. Walters, DPM*, Samuel S. Mendicino, DPM

KEYWORDS

- Posterior tibial tendon dysfunction • Pes planus • Posterior tibial • Foot • Ankle
- Flexor digitorum longus • Flexor digitorum

KEY POINTS

- Isolated soft tissue procedures are generally indicated only in early diagnosis of the flexible adult flatfoot.
- Tendon transfer is not completed to restore full strength to the posterior tibial tendon but to oppose the deforming force of peroneus brevis.
- The advancements in knowledge of the pathomechanics of the deformity have modified the role that soft tissue repair plays in surgical treatment, but the importance of soft tissue restoration in flatfoot repair should not be overlooked.

INTRODUCTION

Classically, adult posterior tibial (PT) tendon dysfunction (PTTD) was considered primarily a tendon rupture and was treated as such with soft tissue repair alone. The understanding that PTTD involves more than simply an inflammatory condition or tendon rupture but also a muscle imbalance, leading to a flatfoot, osteoarthritis, and peritalar subluxation, led to surgeons advocating osseous procedures as well. The advancements in knowledge of the pathomechanics of the deformity have modified the role that soft tissue repair plays in surgical treatment, but the importance of soft tissue restoration in flatfoot repair should not be overlooked.

PT TENDON TENOLYSIS AND AUGMENTATION

Originally, this condition was considered primarily a tendon rupture, and the same principles were applied to PTTD that were used for other tendon injuries. Tenolysis with synovectomy may be helpful in patients with pain and swelling of the PT tendon who fail to respond to conservative and nonoperative management and have not

Relationship Disclosure: The authors have no disclosures to report.
West Houston Medical and Surgical Residency Program PMSR/RRA, West Houston Medical Center, 12121 Richmond Avenue, Suite 417, Houston, TX 77082, USA
* Corresponding author.
E-mail address: jeremylwalters@gmail.com

experienced an acute rupture or tear (**Fig. 1**).[1–3] Teasdall and Johnson[1] reported 74% success with a 30-month follow-up but believed debridement alone should be reserved for patients without a progressive deformity. Funk and colleagues[4] looked at tenosynovectomy with and without repair of a split tendon tear and found 89% of patients with absent or minor pain.

For the patient with an acute midsubstance rupture, primary repair with or without soft tissue support should be considered (**Fig. 2**).[5] In the longitudinal tear with minimal lengthening or weakness, tendon debulking with entubulation may be performed (**Fig. 3**). This treatment may be further supported by tendon augmentation, transfer, or the use of orthobiological substitutes (**Fig. 4**).

FLEXOR DIGITORUM LONGUS TRANSFER

Flexor digitorum longus (FDL) tendon transfer has long been advocated in the treatment of Johnson and Strom stage 2 adult flatfoot deformity and is performed after primary tendon repair.[6–10] For an FDL transfer to be the most effective, or functional, 2 important patient characteristics need to exist. First, a flexible deformity must be present. The FDL tendon cannot overcome a fixed hindfoot valgus if less than 15° of subtalar inversion is present. Second, a patient needs to show a minimum adduction to lock the midtarsal joint, thus permitting heel raise. The choice of FDL as the tendon transfer for PTTD is logical for many reasons. The FDL originates from the posterior tibia adjacent to the PT tendon, without any vital neurovascular structures from the flexor retinaculum to the navicular tuberosity (**Fig. 5**). The FDL also constitutes an in-phase transfer, which is always preferable in tendon transfers.[11]

Sammarco and colleagues[12] and others have advocated use of the flexor hallucis longus (FHL) in lieu of the FDL, because the FHL is more tendinous, closer in strength

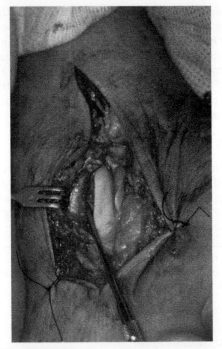

Fig. 1. Tenosynovitis of the PT tendon.

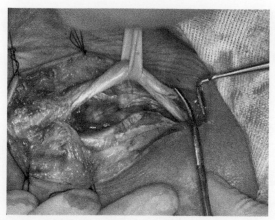

Fig. 2. Midsubstance tear of the PT tendon.

to the PT tendon, and, with its proximity to the sustentaculum tali, could aid in relocating the talus if sutured properly.[13,14] Silver and colleagues[15] reported that the FDL is approximately 30% the strength of the PT tendon and the FHL is twice as strong as the FDL. It is partly because of Silver's work that it was questioned whether the FDL was strong enough to compensate for the loss of PT tendon function and whether a stronger muscle such as the FHL was a better tendon for selection.

However, the goal of the tendon transfer is to help counteract the deforming force of the peroneus brevis (PB), which is 42% as strong as the PT tendon. Taking into

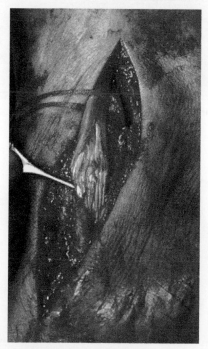

Fig. 3. Longitudinal tear with functional weakening.

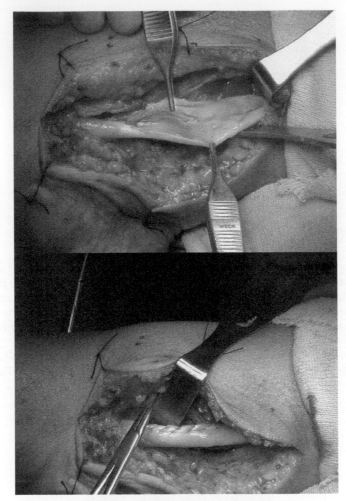

Fig. 4. PT tendon debulking and entubulation.

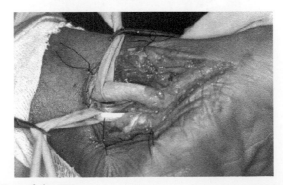

Fig. 5. Identification of the FDL.

account the loss of 1 strength grade with transfer, the FDL transfer is deficient approximately 47% in opposing the PB. For the FDL transfer alone to be strong enough, there must exist 20% residual PT tendon strength, or the PT tendon can use up to 80% of its strength, and an FDL transfer alone provides enough opposition to the PB. This reduction in strength may also explain the return of supinatory power without arch restoration. Given the potential hallux complications when sacrificing the FHL, our preferred technique is to use the FDL tendon for transfer and augmentation and attach the distal FDL stump to the FHL to give plantarflexor stability to the lesser digits.

With proper procedure selection, the outcomes of an FDL transfer in a stage 2 deformity are reliable and predictable. Fayazi and colleagues,[16] Jahss,[17] Mann and Thompson,[7] Shereff,[9] Gazdag and Cracchiolo,[19] and Feldman and colleagues[18] all have reported good to excellent results.

Contraindications include symptomatic arthritis of the talonavicular, subtalar, or calcaneocuboid joints as well as fixed forefoot varus or completely ruptured PT tendon.

PLANTAR CALCANEONAVICULAR LIGAMENT PLICATION AND RECONSTRUCTION

Gazdag and Cracchiolo[19] reported an 81% incidence of plantar calcaneonavicular ligament attenuation in patients with PTTD. Loss of the plantar calcaneonavicular ligament alone does not produce a flatfoot deformity but loss of the ligament with repeated loading does create a deformity; magnetic resonance imaging studies have shown that the deltoid ligament is a major contributor as well in the pathophysiology.[20,21]

It is routine for many surgeons to plicate the ligament as part of an FDL transfer, but Mann[10] found that ligament plication does not correlate with improved results, likely because of a long-standing degenerative process of the ligament. Mann advocated that emphasis should be placed on reconstruction, whether autogenous or allograft reconstruction. Reconstruction of the calcaneonavicular ligament has been performed using tibialis anterior tendon, peroneus longus tendon, PB tendon, and allograft tissue.[21–23] Recently, the InternalBrace ligament augmentation repair (Arthrex, Naples, FL, USA) was introduced with FiberTape technology. It is recommended that the InternalBrace should not be used in isolation but in addition to calcaneal osteotomies or cuneiform osteotomy. It offers similar benefits over autogenous grafting to allograft tendon. No studies have been reported on the use of InternalBrace for calcaneonavicular ligament repair, because the current literature has been devoted toward studying its use in lateral ankle instability.

Although often discussed, especially in regards to biomechanics of the flatfoot deformity; there exist few quality studies on calcaneonavicular ligament reconstruction. If one was to perform a reconstruction, use of allograft tendon would eliminate possibility of donor site pain that can occur with autogenous grafting. No literature was found that evaluated outcomes of ligament reconstruction, isolated or in combination with other transfers or procedures.

COBB TENDON TRANSFER

Cobb tendon transfer was initially described by Helal in 1990,[24] who used the medial half of the tibialis anterior tendon to bridge a defect or as augmentation of a primary repair. Once PT tendon repair and any osseous realignment procedures have been performed, a 2-cm incision is deepened at the myotendinous junction of the anterior tibial tendon, and the medial aspect of the tendon identified and harvested through the distal incision, thus preserving the attachment of the muscle (**Fig. 6**).[24] The tendon is used to bridge a deficit or augment a primary repair by transferring to the posterior

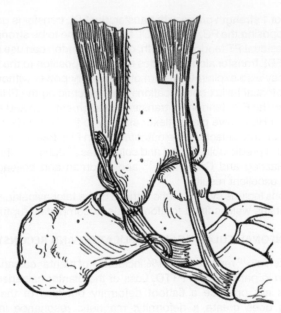

Fig. 6. The Cobb procedure.

compartment and attaching it through a drill hole in the medial cuneiform.[24] Weil and colleagues[25] reported excellent results using the Cobb procedure in stage 2 PTTD. This procedure is more consistent with a soft tissue augmentation procedure than a true tendon transfer. It is our opinion that although this is a relative simple and easy to perform procedure, it should be left to historical anecdote. Sacrificing the tibialis anterior tendon, which not only weakens the tendon at a minimum of 1 grade but also sacrifices another major inverter/adductor of the foot, for a tendon augmentation is difficult to rationalize on a biomechanics level.

SUMMARY

PTTD is a complex multifaceted disease, which if misdiagnosed can quickly progress to a very painful and severe condition. Early recognition is important, and soft tissue repair, if performed in the early stages, may prevent aggressive surgical procedures. Outside stage 1 and early stage 2, the role of isolated soft tissue procedures is limited and should generally be combined with other adjunctive osseous procedures.

REFERENCES

1. Teasdall R, Johnson KA. Surgical treatment of stage 1 posterior tibial tendon dysfunction. Foot Ankle Int 1994;12:646–8.
2. Trevino S, Gould N, Korson R. Surgical treatment of stenosing tenosynovitis at the ankle. Foot Ankle 1981;2:37–45.
3. Williams R. Chronic non-specific tendovaginitis of tibialis posterior. J Bone Joint Surg Br 1963;45:542–5.
4. Funk DA, Cass JR, Johnson KA. Acquired adult flat foot secondary to posterior tibial tendon pathology. J Bone Joint Surg Am 1986;68:95–101.
5. Gould J. Direct repair of the posterior tibial tendon. Foot Ankle Clin 1974;2: 275–9.

6. Hansen S, Clark W. Tendon transfer to augment the weakened tibialis posterior mechanism. J Am Podiatr Med Assoc 1988;78:399–402.
7. Mann RA, Thompson FM. Rupture of the posterior tibial tendon causing flatfoot. J Bone Joint Surg Am 1985;67:556.
8. Mendicino S, Quinn M. Tibialis posterior dysfunction: an overview with a surgical case report using a flexor tendon transfer. J Foot Surg 1989;28:154–7.
9. Shereff M. Treatment of ruptured posterior tibial tendon with direct repair and FDL tenodesis. Foot Ankle Clin 1997;2:281–96.
10. Mann RA. Posterior tibial tendon dysfunction treatment by flexor digitorum longus transfer. Foot Ankle Clin 2001;6:77–87.
11. Mann RA, Coughlin MJ. Surgery of the foot and ankle. 6th edition. St Louis (MO): Mosby; 1993.
12. Sammarco GJ, Hockenbury RT. Treatment of stage II posterior tibial tendon dysfunction with flexor hallucis longus transfer and medial displacement calcaneal osteotomy. Foot Ankle Int 2001;22(4):305–12.
13. Mulier T, Rummens E, Dereymaeker G. Risk of neurovascular injuries in flexor hallucis longus tendon transfers: an anatomic cadaver study. Foot Ankle Int 2007; 28(8):910–5.
14. Goldner JL, Keats PK, Bassett FH. Progressive talipes equinovalgus due to trauma or degeneration of the posterior tibial tendon and medial plantar ligaments. Orthop Clin North Am 1974;5(1):39–51.
15. Silver RL, Garza J, Rang M. The myth of muscle balance. J Bone Joint Surg Br 1985;3(67):432–7.
16. Fayazi AH, Nguyen HV, Juliano PJ. Intermediate term follow-up of calcaneal osteotomy and flexor digitorum longus transfer for treatment of posterior tibial tendon dysfunction. Foot Ankle Int 2002;23(12):1107–11.
17. Jahss MH. Spontaneous rupture of the tibialis posterior tendon: clinical findings, tenographic studies and a new technique of repair. Foot Ankle 1982;3(3):158–66.
18. Feldman NJ, Oloff LM, Schulhofer SD. In situ tibialis posterior to flexor digitorum longus tendon transfer for tibialis posterior tendon dysfunction: a simplified surgical approach with outcome of 11 patients. J Foot Ankle Surg 2001;40(1):2–7.
19. Gazdag AE, Cracchiolo A. Rupture of the posterior tibial tendon: evaluation of injury of the spring ligament and clinical assessment of tendon transfer and ligament repair. J Bone Joint Surg Am 1997;79:675–81.
20. Deland JT, Sung IH, Potter H. Posterior tibial tendon dysfunction: which ligaments are involved?. Presented at summer meeting Puerto Rico: American Orthopaedic Foot and Ankle Society; 1999.
21. Thordarson DB, Schmotzer H, Chon J. Reconstruction with tenodesis in an adult flat foot model. J Bone Joint Surg Am 1995;77:1557–64.
22. Choi K, Lee S, Otis JC, et al. Anatomical reconstruction of the spring ligament using peroneus longus tendon graft. Foot Ankle 2003;24:430–6.
23. Deland JT, Annoczky S, Thompson FM. Adult acquired flatfoot deformity at the talonavicular joint: reconstruction of the spring ligament in an in vitro model. Foot Ankle Int 1992;13:327–32.
24. Helal B. Cobb repair for tibialis posterior tendon rupture. J Foot Surg 1990;29: 349–52.
25. Weil LS Jr, Benton-Weil W, Borrelli AH, et al. Outcomes for surgical correction for stages 2 and 3 tibialis posterior dysfunction. J Foot Ankle Surg 1998;37:467–71.

Is Advanced Imaging Necessary Before Surgical Repair

John M. Baca, DPM[a],*, Colin Zdenek, DPM[a],
Alan R. Catanzariti, DPM[a], Robert W. Mendicino, DPM[b,c]

KEYWORDS

- Imaging • Ultrasound • MRI • Posterior tibial tendon dysfunction
- Adult acquired flatfoot

KEY POINTS

- Plain-film weight-bearing radiographs continue to be the mainstay for initial imaging of structural deformity in patients with adult acquired flatfoot (AAFF).
- Although AAFF is frequently diagnosed based on incisive clinical acumen, magnetic resonance imaging (MRI) can provide abundant evidence regarding the health and quality of hindfoot articulations and soft tissues.
- The complex nature of AAFF entails insufficiency of numerous structures in addition to the posterior tibial tendon. Underlying deficiency of the deltoid complex and/or spring ligament can be more thoroughly assessed with MRI.
- In the appropriate setting with trained personnel, ultrasound can be a powerful and inexpensive imaging modality to appraise the pertinent soft tissue structures associated with AAFF.

Posterior tibial tendon (PTT) dysfunction (tendinitis, tendinosis, or rupture) and adult acquired flatfoot deformity can manifest with a wide array of bony and soft tissue abnormalities visible on plain radiographs, ultrasound, and magnetic resonance imaging (MRI). Imaging abnormalities include various combinations of malalignment, anatomic variants, and enthesopathic and tendinopathic changes.[1–3] A thorough understanding of differences between anatomic and pathologic presentations of structures in various imaging modalities is an essential tool for clinical and surgical planning.

[a] Division of Foot & Ankle Surgery, West Penn Hospital, 4800 Friendship Avenue, Pittsburgh, PA 15224, USA; [b] Department of Orthopoedics, OhioHealth Orthopedic Surgeons, 4343 All Seasons Drive, Suite 140, Hilliard, OH 43026, USA; [c] Foot & Ankle Surgical Residency, West Penn Hospital, 4800 Friendship Avenue, Pittsburgh, PA 15224, USA
* Corresponding author. West Penn Allegheny Health System, 320 East North Avenue, Pittsburgh, PA 15212.
E-mail address: jbaca@wpahs.org

Clin Podiatr Med Surg 31 (2014) 357–362
http://dx.doi.org/10.1016/j.cpm.2014.03.010
0891-8422/14/$ – see front matter © 2014 Elsevier Inc. All rights reserved.

podiatric.theclinics.com

PLAIN RADIOGRAPHS

Abnormal bony position observed with plain radiographs may give clues to long-standing insufficiency of the PTT. Malalignment and angular deformity on radiographs often correlate to soft tissue abnormalities identified on ultrasound and MRI.[1] Three weight-bearing views (lateral, anteroposterior, medial oblique) of the foot are generally necessary to evaluate for signs of PTT dysfunction. Ankle views are necessary to evaluate for valgus deformity, especially with advanced deformity (**Fig. 1**). Additional hindfoot alignment views (calcaneal axial, long-leg axial) may be beneficial to ascertain the frontal plane relationship of the tibia, talus, and calcaneus (**Fig. 2**).

Flattening of the plantar arch on a lateral weight-bearing view may be observed through evaluating the calcaneal inclination angle. Although variation normally ranges from 11° to 38°, it is considered low when it is less than 20°.[4,5] Attenuation and weakness of the surrounding supporting soft tissue structures may lead to increased talar declination of the long axis of the talus below the long axis of the navicular. Talar declination, normally 21°(±4°), is measured using the lateral talar axis and the weight-bearing surface.[1,4]

Secondary to the unopposed force of the peroneal tendons, mainly the peroneus brevis, hindfoot valgus and forefoot abduction may be appreciated.[5] Greater than a 6° angulation of the long axis of the calcaneus away from midline relative to the long axis of the tibia in the frontal plane defines hindfoot valgus.[4,6] Uncovering of the head of the talus as the navicular moves away from midline in the transverse plane is the result of forefoot abduction. Talar head uncovering is considered abnormal if more than 15% of the head is exposed.[6]

Hypertrophic change and bony irregularity may also be noted at the navicular attachment of the PTT, which suggests enthesopathy.[1] Another sign of posterior tibialis tendinopathy is a tibial spur, which may be visible adjacent to the tendon in the retromalleolar groove.[1,6] Congenital navicular abnormalities may also predispose patients to tendinopathy. A true accessory navicular is present in approximatley 4%

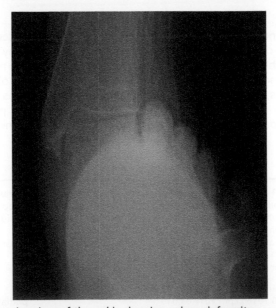

Fig. 1. Anteroposterior view of the ankle showing valgus deformity.

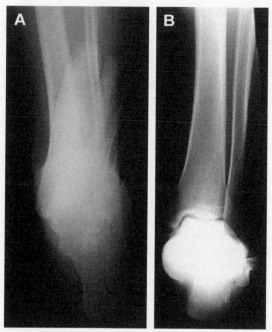

Fig. 2. (*A*) Long-leg axial view. (*B*) Hindfoot alignment view.

of the population[7]; however, accessory naviculars are present in a much higher percentage of patients with posterior tibialis tendon disorders.[8] Accessory navicular variants (types 2 and 3) are visible on MRI similar to plain radiographs.[1]

ULTRASOUND

Ultrasound is an inexpensive and easily accessible tool for evaluating the PTT and other relevant soft tissue structures. The tendon course is relatively superficial and amendable to sonographic evaluation.[1] Unlike MRI, ultrasound allows for dynamic assessment of tendon function and evaluation of focal areas of tenderness.[1,3] However, one drawback is that ultrasound evaluation is highly technician dependent and may be more reliable with musculoskeletal trained sonographers and radiologists.

Posterior tibial tendon dysfunction has been described most frequently at its insertion onto the navicular tubercle (inframalleolar), and occasionally adjacent to the medial malleolus (retromalleolar), and may be caused by increased friction in this area.[3,7,9–11] Jain and colleagues,[3] however, also described tendon abnormalities above the border of the medial malleolus and adjacent to the flexor retinaculum (supramalleolar). Ultrasound was used to assess tendon abnormalities in this area, because MRI often does not evaluate the tendon this proximally. The tendon was evaluated for hallmark signs of tenosynovitis (fluid collection, hyperemia, and focal or diffuse tendon sheath thickening) using ultrasound in each of the 3 generalized regions previously defined. Tendon abnormalities were then classified as either grade 1 (tenosynovitis), 2 (partial tear), or 3 (complete tear).[7,9] Although only 5.1% of their study patients had supramalleolar abnormalities, the investigators found more severe grades of tear and increased prevalence of tenosynovitis in these patients.[3] When compared with MRI, Nallamshetty and colleagues[7] found ultrasound findings to be concordant with those of MRI in most cases. Ultrasound was found to be less sensitive than MRI (69% vs 73%) in identifying posterior tendon abnormalities; however, because the diagnosis of PTT dysfunction remains primarily clinical, they found that these discrepancies did not affect clinical management.[3,10] Dynamic evaluation of the posterior tendon may be able to identify transient subluxation or dislocation from the retromalleolar groove.[1]

The spring ligament can also be evaluated using ultrasound passing between the sustentaculum tali and the navicular. Absence of this structure deep to the PTT would suggest a tear. Harish and colleagues[12] showed that ultrasound findings were equivalent to MR findings in 94% of cases in identifying spring ligament abnormalities. The sinus tarsi may also be visualized with ultrasound at the anteroinferior tip of the lateral malleolus. Edema in this area would be suggested by signal heterogeneity.[1]

MRI

Magnetic resonance imaging is the gold standard for assessing disorders of the PTT and other associated soft tissue structures. Magnetic resonance imaging also allows evaluation of bony edema compared with plain radiographs and ultrasound.[1,6,12] The PTT is normally ovoid in shape and approximately double the size of the nearby flexor digitorum longus.[1] As it courses distally, a normal trace amount of fluid in the sheath may be present if it seems to be less than 2 mm in thickness and is not circumferential in nature.[6]

The surrounding tendon sheath usually extends distally to within 1 to 2 cm of the navicular insertion. Therefore, if fluid is observed around the distal segment of the tendon, one should suspect metaplastic synovitis rather than tenosynovitis.[6] Paratendinitis is used to describe synovitis, or fluid, around the tendon with no evidence of a tear.[13] A type 1 partial tear should be suspected if the tendon is hypertrophied and rounded, increased intrasubstance signal is present, or longitudinal tears are observed. Type 2 tears would consist of tendon atrophy to a diameter less than that of the adjacent flexor digitorum longus. Type 3 tears with complete tendon absence may be seen with or without and empty tendon sheath.[1]

The spring ligament can also be visualized in great detail using MRI.[12,14] Gazdag and Cracchiolo[15] stressed the importance of evaluating the spring ligament complex, because they noted the involvement of the superomedial portion of the ligament in most patients treated surgically.[16] The spring ligament should be seen as a hypointense signal band bounded by 4 anatomic landmarks: sustentaculum tali, talar head, navicular, and posterior tibial tendon. It is normally surrounded by fat but may contact nearby bone or tendon. The course of the ligament may be difficult to follow as it courses between the sustentaculum tali and the navicular if it is not completely in the transverse plane of the MRI scan. In this case, the addition of ultrasound may aid in surgical planning. Lack of continuity, signal abnormalities, or surrounding edema may indicate spring ligament compromise.[1]

Magnetic resonance imaging is also useful for evaluating other ligamentous structures in the foot and ankle.[14,16,17] Deland and colleagues[16] showed that PTT insufficiency was most commonly associated with damage to the superomedial portion and the inferior calcaneonavicular portion of the spring ligament. The superomedial portion of the spring ligament is the largest and strongest structure, and includes the medial talonavicular joint capsule.[18] This superior portion contains both fibrous and fibrocartilaginous tissue, which likely results from talar head compression on the posterior tibial tendon. The inferior portion is narrow and entirely fibrous in nature. Because of its common involvement in PTT insufficiency, the spring ligament is the one ligament that should be protected or surgically reconstructed.[16]

The interosseous talocalcaneal ligament was also commonly affected, with grade II, III, or IV tears seen in 48% of study patients.[16] In addition, Donovan and Rosenberg[19] showed that extraarticular lateral hindfoot impingement (chiefly talocalcaneal-subfibular) was associated with advanced-stage PTT tears.

The authors consider MRI in evaluating the deltoid ligament in late-stage III deformity. They consider deltoid repair and/or medial displacement calcaneal osteotomy when evidence of a partial rupture or attenuation is seen on MRI. Song and colleagues,[20] when reviewing tensile forces through the deltoid ligament with PTT dysfunction, have recommended MRI evaluation before flatfoot reconstruction.

Unlike adults, adolescents may not demonstrate all or any of the late-stage MRI findings discussed previously. Wong and Griffith[21] hypothesized that the navicular tuberosity pain commonly experienced with the adolescent flexible flatfoot was associated with navicular insertional posterior tibial tendon enthesopathy. Nearly 42% of their study patients manifested MRI findings of thickening of the PTT insertion, accessory navicular marrow edema, navicular tuberosity marrow edema, or contrast enhancement of the PTT insertion site. These findings might explain the origin of adolescent flatfoot pain, and early identification and treatment could prevent progression.

IS ADVANCED IMAGING NECESSARY?

Magnetic resonance imaging and diagnostic ultrasound provide unique information regarding soft tissue structures in PTT dysfunction; however, the authors question the necessity of these diagnostic tests. Recent classification systems used to select surgical procedures that address the various components of PTT dysfunction depend on clinical assessment and radiographic findings. Although these test results may provide some prognostic information, they are not necessary to develop a surgical plan, because direct inspection and functional assessment of the PTT will dictate decision making.

SUMMARY

Posterior tibial tendon dysfunction is a progressive disease that alters soft tissue structures and osseous alignment. Evaluation with plain radiographs, ultrasound, and MRI may be beneficial for evaluating osseous and soft tissue abnormalities but is also helpful in assessing bony changes and malalignment.[1] Advanced imaging to evaluate soft tissue structures is not always necessary.

REFERENCES

1. Kong A, Van Der Vleit A. Imaging of tibialis posterior dysfunction. Br J Radiol 2008;81:826–36.
2. Chhabra A, Soldatos T, Chalian M, et al. 3-Tesla magnetic resonance imaging evolution of posterior tibial tendon dysfunction with relevance to clinical stages. J Foot Ankle Surg 2011;50:320–8.
3. Jain NB, Omar I, Kelikian AS, et al. Prevalence of and factors associated with posterior tibial tendon pathology on sonographic assessment. PM R 2011;3: 998–1004.
4. Weissman SD. Radiology of the foot. Baltimore (MD): Williams & Wilkins; 1989.
5. Berquist TH, editor. Radiology of the foot and ankle. Philadelphia: Lippincott, Williams & Wilkins; 2000.
6. Schweitzer ME, Karasick D. MR imaging of disorders of the posterior tibialis tendon. AJR Am J Roentgenol 2000;175:627–35.

7. Nallamshetty L, Nazarian LN, Schweitzer ME, et al. Evaluation of posterior tibial pathology: comparison of sonography and MR imaging. Skeletal Radiol 2005; 34:375–80.
8. Schweitzer ME, Caccese R, Karasick D. Posterior tibial tendon tears: utility of secondary signs for MR imaging diagnosis. Radiology 1993;188:655–9.
9. Conti SF. Posterior tibial tendon problems in athletes. Orthop Clin North Am 1994; 25:109–21.
10. Johnson KA, Strom DE. Tibialis posterior tendon dysfunction. Clin Orthop Relat Res 1989;(239):196–206.
11. Rosenberg ZS, Beltran J, Benicardino JT. From the RSNA Refresher Courses. Radiological Society of North America. MR imaging of the ankle and foot. Radiographics 2000;20:S130–79.
12. Harish S, Kumbhare D, O'Neill J, et al. Comparison of sonography and magnetic resonance imaging for spring ligament abnormalities: preliminary study. J Ultrasound Med 2008;27:1145–52.
13. Premkumar A, Perry M, Dwyer A, et al. Sonography and MR imaging of posterior tibial tendinopathy. AJR Am J Roentgenol 2002;178:223–32.
14. Yao L, Gentilli A, Cracchiolo A. MR imaging findings in spring ligament insufficiency. Skeletal Radiol 1999;28:245–50.
15. Gazdag AR, Cracchiolo A III. Rupture of the posterior tibial tendon. Evaluation of injury of the spring ligament and clinical assessment of tendon transfer and ligament repair. J Bone Joint Surg Am 1997;79:675–81.
16. Deland JT, de Asla RJ, Sung IH, et al. Posterior tibial tendon insufficiency: which ligaments are involved? Foot Ankle Int 2005;26:427–35.
17. Timins ME. MR imaging of the foot and ankle. Foot Ankle Clin 2000;5:83–101.
18. Davis WH, Sobel M, DiCarlo EF, et al. Gross, histological, and microvascular anatomy and biomechanical testing of the spring ligament complex. Foot Ankle Int 1996;17:95–102.
19. Donovan A, Rosenberg ZS. Extraarticular lateral hindfoot impingement with posterior tibial tendon tear: MRI correlation. AJR Am J Roentgenol 2009;193: 672–8.
20. Song SJ, Lee S, O'Malley MJ, et al. Deltoid ligament strain after correction of acquired flatfoot deformity by triple arthrodesis. Foot Ankle Int 2000;21(7):573–7.
21. Wong MW, Griffith JF. Magnetic resonance imaging in adolescent painful flexible flatfoot. Foot Ankle Int 2009;30:303–8.

Procedure Selection for the Flexible Adult Acquired Flatfoot Deformity

Matthew J. Hentges, DPM[a], Kyle R. Moore, DPM[a],
Alan R. Catanzariti, DPM[a,*], Richard Derner, DPM[b]

KEYWORDS

- Posterior tibial tendon dysfunction • Adult acquired flatfoot
- Posterior calcaneal displacement osteotomy • Lateral column lengthening
- Flexor digitorum longus tendon transfer

KEY POINTS

- Posterior tibial tendon (PTT) dysfunction (PTTD) is the most common cause of adult acquired flatfoot. Failure of the static constraints of the medial column, followed by failure of the PTT, leads to this deformity.
- Equinus deformity of the posterior muscle group is often present and must be addressed.
- The flexible (or nonfixed) adult acquired flatfoot is managed by selective use of calcaneal osteotomies, tendon transfers, and posterior muscle group lengthening.
- Arthrodesis of nonessential joints of the medial column is used to assist in complete reduction of the foot deformity.
- Early identification and aggressive management of the flexible adult acquired flatfoot is important in preventing progression of the deformity, adaptation of the osseous and soft-tissue structures, end-stage arthritis, and ankle malalignment.

INTRODUCTION

Adult acquired flatfoot (AAFF) is a common musculoskeletal condition encountered by foot and ankle surgeons. There have been more articles published in peer-reviewed journals in the past 10 years relating to the AAFF than virtually any other topic. Nebulous treatment options have become more formalized, especially with surgery, due to the improved classification systems and advances in technology. However, there remain regional differences among surgeons in the management of the nonfixed AAFF.

Disclosures: The authors have no disclosures related to the production of this article.
[a] Division of Foot and Ankle Surgery, West Penn Hospital, Allegheny Health Network, 4800 Friendship Avenue, Pittsburgh, PA 15224, USA; [b] Private Practice, Associated Foot and Ankle Centers of Northern Virginia, 1721 Financial Loop, Lake Ridge, VA 22192, USA
* Corresponding author.
E-mail address: acatanzariti@faiwp.com

AAFF is a progressive deformity characterized by collapse of the medial longitudinal arch and dysfunction or insufficiency of the posteromedial and medial soft-tissue constraints of the ankle and hindfoot. The cause of this deformity is most commonly associated with PTTD; however, it can also be secondary to inflammatory arthritis or trauma.

In their classic article, Johnson and Strom[1] described 3 stages of PTTD beginning with painful synovitis progressing to a nonfixed flatfoot deformity and ending with a fixed arthritic flatfoot. This classification system was later modified by Myerson[2] to include a fourth stage encompassing deformity of the ankle. Weinraub and Heilala[3] created a classification system and an algorithmic surgical approach for the treatment of AAFF. This classification system combined both osseous and soft-tissue components into a staging (soft-tissue component) and grading (osseous component) system. Selection of surgical procedures was based off of this combined staging and grading system. A recent classification published by Haddad and colleagues[4] divides stage II into 5 different subcategories (A–E) (**Table 1**). This article focuses on the

Table 1
Comparison of classification systems for adult acquired flatfoot

Classifications for Adult Acquired Flatfoot Deformity	Johnson & Strom,[1] 1989	Weinraub & Heilala,[3] 2000	Haddad et al,[4] 2011
Stage I	PT tenosynovitis, no clinical foot deformity	I A—acute posterior tibial (PT) tendonitis, no deformity I B—acute PT tendonitis, reducible (nonfixed) deformity I C—acute PT tendonitis, rigid deformity	I A—inflammatory disease (ie, rheumatoid arthritis) I B—partial PTT tear, no clinical deformity I C—partial PTT tear, slight hindfoot valgus
Stage II	Reducible hindfoot valgus	II A—PT tendinosis, medial soft-tissue attenuation, no deformity II B—PT tendinosis, medial soft-tissue attenuation, reducible (nonfixed) deformity II C—PT tendinosis, medial soft-tissue attenuation, rigid deformity	II A—reducible hindfoot valgus II B—flexible forefoot supination II C—fixed forefoot supination II D—forefoot abduction II E—medial ray instability
Stage III	Rigid hindfoot valgus	III A—advanced PTT attenuation or rupture, no deformity III B—advanced PTT attenuation or rupture, reducible (nonfixed) deformity III C—advanced PTT attenuation or rupture, rigid deformity	III A—rigid hindfoot valgus III B—rigid hindfoot valgus, forefoot abduction and/or sagittal plane instability
Stage IV	Valgus deformity of the ankle (added by Myerson)[2]		IV A—flexible ankle valgus IV B—rigid ankle valgus

pathoanatomy, diagnosis, and current surgical management of the nonfixed AAFF based on these contemporary classifications.

PATHOANATOMY

The pertinent anatomy of the nonfixed AAFF includes not only the PTT but also the spring ligament, deltoid ligament, the articulations of the tritarsal complex (talonavicular joint, subtalar joint, and calcaneal-cuboid joint), and the medial column (naviculo-cuneiform joint and first tarsometatarsal joint). The PTT takes its origin from the posterior aspect of the tibia, fibula, and interosseous membrane. The tendon courses posterior to the medial malleolus and inserts into the navicular tuberosity and multiple additional insertions across the plantar aspect of the midfoot.[5] The vascular supply to the PTT consists of branches of the posterior tibial artery. Proximally, muscular branches feed the tendon. Distally, periosteal branches feed the tendon. A watershed area, or zone of hypovascularity, has been identified in the retromalleolar region of the PTT, which often corresponds to one of the sites of degenerative changes within the tendon.[6] The degenerative changes within the tendon may be the result of repetitive microtrauma or compromised repair response due to the limited vascular supply.[7]

The spring ligament complex extends from the anterior margin of the sustentaculum tali to the plantar medial aspect of the navicular and cradles the plantar medial aspect of the talar head.[7] This ligamentous complex comprises a superomedial and inferior calcaneonavicular ligament. The superomedial calcaneonavicular ligament is commonly involved in the AAFF deformity and is often found intraoperatively to be attenuated or torn.[8]

The deltoid ligament complex has multiple components, both superficial and deep. It blends distally with the spring ligament complex and the talonavicular joint capsule.[7] Attenuation of the deltoid ligament due to long-standing valgus deformity of the hindfoot can lead to valgus tilting of the talus within the ankle mortise, which is the case in stage IV AAFF.

Muscle balance of the lower extremity is altered with dysfunction of the PTT and resultant AAFF. The PTT produces inversion of the hindfoot and locks the midtarsal joint to maintain the medial longitudinal arch and create a rigid lever for push off during normal gait. When the PTT is diseased, it no longer creates an inversion moment on the hindfoot and the peroneus brevis gains a mechanical advantage. The midtarsal joint is then unlocked, and the hindfoot can no longer function as a rigid lever for push off. Moreover, during heel strike, the eccentric contraction of the PTT is limited, thereby increasing the valgus moment of the hindfoot. In combination with an equinus contracture, there is increased stress placed on the medial column of the foot. The repetitive biomechanical alteration in the gait cycle creates progressive midfoot collapse, forefoot abduction, and hindfoot valgus.[9] There are 2 potential mechanical causes of AAFF. First, medial column instability resulting in a forefoot supinatus deformity and a compensatory hindfoot valgus.[7] Second, contracture of the posterior muscle group, either gastrocnemius equinus or gastrocnemius-soleus equinus, results in breakdown of the medial column of the foot, peritalar subluxation, and subfibular impingement due to hindfoot valgus.[6]

DIAGNOSIS OF STAGE II AAFF
Clinical Presentation

Although the clinical diagnosis of AAFF is well understood, the subtleties of stage II flatfoot are less well characterized. Patients typically present with a painful and swollen medial hindfoot and/or ankle. They may relate the pain radiating into the medial arch or proximally into the leg. As the deformity continues to progress, patients may present with lateral hindfoot pain and/or pain in the sinus tarsi region.

Many patients present for evaluation and treatment during their fifth or sixth decade of life. Often, they have had a flatfoot their entire life, and relate a gradual onset of pain over months to years. For those without a congenital flatfoot, they may be able to correlate the decrease in arch height and onset of symptoms. Most patients deny an acute traumatic event; however, some may identify a specific event that preceded the pain and loss of arch height (**Fig. 1**). Standing for extended periods and normal ambulation typically triggers pain in the medial hindfoot and posteromedial ankle. Patients often note dysfunctional gait, with a decreased ability to run and a loss of push off strength.[7] It is important to obtain a detailed history, including trauma to the foot and/or ankle, family history of flatfeet, chronic steroid use, diabetes mellitus, inflammatory arthritides, and smoking. It is also important to identify patients with multiarticular hypermobility, such as Ehlers-Danlos syndrome, as these patients often present similar to PTT dysfunction. Previous attempts at treatment should also be elicited, including both nonoperative and operative interventions.

Clinical Examination

The comprehensive assessment of the patient with symptomatic flatfoot should be firmly rooted in a thorough history and physical examination. Careful attention to complaints such as arch fatigue, ankle discomfort, or proximal lower extremity pain should be noted. It is important to formulate a methodical and systematic approach to examine the patient in a complete yet timely manner. The stepwise progression of PTTD and AAFF has been well documented during the past 2 decades.[1–3,10–12] The distinct clinical features originally proposed by Johnson and Strom[1] have allowed the practitioner to better understand the continuum of PTTD and AAFF.

The flatfoot evaluation includes open kinetic chain examination, static stance weight-bearing examination, and dynamic gait analysis, all of which are frequently

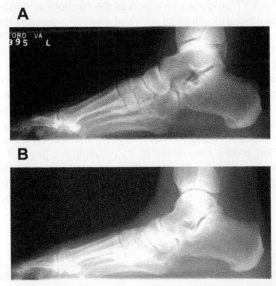

Fig. 1. (*A*) Preinjury and (*B*) postinjury radiographs of a traumatic rupture of the posterior tibial tendon.

supplemented with radiographic imaging. In addition to the above-noted biomechanical and orthopedic examinations, baseline vascular and neurologic status should also be ascertained at the initial office encounter; this is particularly applicable in patients with a high probability of undergoing future surgical intervention. Additional workup may be warranted if vascular deficits are encountered in the elective surgical patient.

The affected lower extremity should be carefully compared with the contralateral limb with the patient seated in the examination chair. A fullness or swelling of the medial arch and ankle can obscure the normal anatomic contours of the tibial malleolus. Subtle erythema or mild callus formation may appear secondary to a partially subluxed talar head or increased medial arch pressure.[6] Palpation of the PTT often elicits tenderness along its course, as well as at the navicular insertion site. Manual strength of the PTT can be easily tested and also should be carefully compared with the unaffected side. Proper positioning of the foot to diminish the contribution of the tibialis anterior tendon is important to fully isolate the strength and function of the PTT.[13] The affected side may appear slightly weak, and/or pain can be provoked if the tendon is palpated while the PTT is being actively contracted. These subtle clues may serve as the few revealing factors to an early-stage deformity as the painful foot may appear structurally similar to the unaffected side when non–weight bearing (**Fig. 2**).

The importance of the medial hindfoot supporting structures, namely, the spring ligament and deltoid ligament, and their role in the valgus hindfoot deformity has been

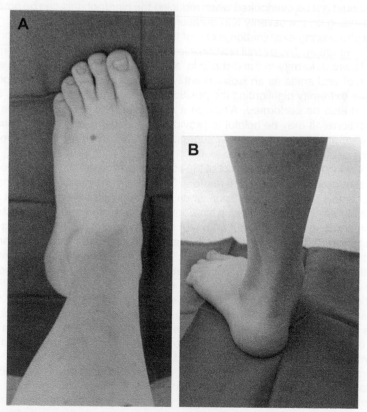

Fig. 2. (*A, B*) Clinical examination of AAFF reveals reducible heel valgus, collapse of medial longitudinal arch, forefoot abduction, forefoot supinatus, and gastrocnemius equinus.

emphasized.[7,14,15] Although it may be difficult to directly isolate these structures during the physical examination, their importance cannot be marginalized during the assessment. Furthermore, concomitant deformities such as hallux valgus can frequently be seen in AAFF and may serve as additional sources of discomfort in the patient with AAFF.[16,17]

Non–weight-bearing joint motion, including that of tibiotalar, subtalar, and midtarsal joints, should also be thoroughly assessed. The definition of a nonfixed flatfoot can be characterized by a reducible hindfoot. This condition is noted on clinical examination through manual manipulation. DiGiovanni and colleagues,[18,19] as well as numerous other investigators, have reported the increased mechanical loads that equinus contracture can produce on the foot and ankle.[20] Thus, ankle joint dorsiflexion necessitates appropriate evaluation and should not be overlooked. A properly performed Silfverskiold examination is crucial not only in revealing the presence of equinus deformity but also in determining the driving component behind reduced ankle joint dorsiflexion (gastrocnemius vs gastrocnemius-soleus vs osseous) and surgical treatment plan.[21]

By firmly stabilizing the calcaneus in a neutral position and applying an abductory force to the lateral forefoot, midtarsal joint excursion can be determined. The degree of abduction and the ability to appreciate a firm end point can provide the examiner beneficial information regarding midtarsal joint stability. One should also examine the reducibility of the medial column and for hypermobility of the first ray. Forefoot supination should not be overlooked when reducing the hindfoot; this can be nonfixed or fixed depending on the severity and duration of the deformity.

The weight-bearing examination is one of the most critical and revealing portions of the AAFF evaluation. The overall relationship of the foot and ankle to the lower leg, as well as intrinsic deformity to the distal tibia, should be noted. One would be remiss to treat the foot and ankle as an isolated entity. Therefore, complete evaluation of the entire lower extremity highlighting the position of the hip girdle, femur, knee, and patella should also be performed. Although it may be somewhat cumbersome for the busy practitioner, it may be helpful to provide examination garments or request that patients wear short pants to uncover suprastructural deformities that can strongly influence the pedal architecture.

When viewing the posterior aspect of the affected lower extremity, the forefoot often appears abducted in relation to the rearfoot. This condition predisposes the patient to the often quoted "too many toes" sign when compared with the contralateral side.[1] A mild to moderate increase in valgus hindfoot position is often present, which should reduce on rising up on the balls of both feet simultaneously. While instructing the patient to lightly stabilize himself or herself on a flat wall or table, the practitioner should attempt to perform the "single heel rise test," as this maneuver is often positive in patients with PTT. When inflammation and/or attenuation of the tendon is present, rising onto the forefoot may be painful or even impossible to perform.[1–3,6,7,10–13,15,22] A dysfunctional PTT is unable to provide an effective supinatory moment to stabilize the midtarsal joint, and the observer can appreciate instability in the arch as the patient attempts to rise up on the toes on the affected foot. Even if the patient is able to perform this maneuver on the initial effort, multiple repeated attempts at heel rise often worsen medial ankle and/or arch discomfort.[2,12]

Hintermann and Gachter[23] described the "first metatarsal rise test" as another sensitive examination to appraise the function of the PTT. This evaluation entails having the patient stand with equally distributed weight on both feet and the examiner passively moving the affected hindfoot into a varus position. In the case of a dysfunctional PTT, the first metatarsal head rises from the weight-bearing surface. Conversely, if the tibialis posterior tendon is functioning normally, the patient is able to keep the first metatarsal in contact with the floor.

The true extent of their pain and discomfort can typically be appreciated as the patient with symptomatic AAFF is asked to walk barefoot across the floor. The gait analysis may expose an antalgic limp that can be coupled with more proximal postural symptoms. The patient may seem to remain in stance phase longer on the affected foot as heel rise occurs later in the gait cycle. Dynamic side-by-side comparison of both feet may reveal a noticeable loss of arch height and increased abduction when compared with the unaffected side. When underlying equinus deformity exists, the examiner may note additional proximal compensatory mechanisms such as genu recurvatum, lumbar lordosis, and forward postural position.[22]

Radiographic Examination

Standard weight-bearing radiographs consisting of anteroposterior (AP) foot, lateral foot, and AP ankle projections should be obtained for both lower extremities (**Fig. 3**). These radiographs warrant careful review for additional pathologic conditions, such as coalitions or neoplastic changes, and positional analysis should be carefully correlated with the clinical examination findings. The aberrant radiographic angles frequently seen in AAFF may be subtle in certain patients, and having contralateral films of the uninvolved foot is helpful in uncovering mild structural changes. In addition, hindfoot alignment and long leg calcaneal axial views may also provide useful information in this patient population.

Abnormal angles on the AP foot projection that are frequently encountered in the AAFF patient include a decreased talonavicular congruency, increased cuboid abduction angle, increased talocalcaneal angle (Kite angle), and increased talo-first metatarsal angle. Lateral foot radiographs can reveal an abnormally decreased calcaneal inclination angle, increased talar declination angle, anterior displacement of the cyma line, decreased medial cuneiform-fifth metatarsal distance, and increased talo-first metatarsal angle (Meary angle).[2,6,7,22–24] Previous studies have shown that the talo-first metatarsal angle is a valuable radiographic identifier of adult flatfoot, and both medial cuneiform-fifth metatarsal distance and calcaneal inclination angle have good interobserver reliability for analyzing the deformity.[24] Finally, although it is much less of a concern in the patient with nonfixed AAFF, ankle valgus has been listed as a potential sequela of end-stage PTTD. For this reason, AP ankle films have become a routine part of the "flatfoot series" radiographs to assess for the presence of this deformity.

Assessment of frontal plane deformity of the hindfoot is an important aspect of the radiographic examination. Special radiographic views, such as hindfoot alignment and long leg calcaneal axial, allow for evaluation of malalignment of the hindfoot relative to the leg.[25,26] These specialized radiographic views allow for assessment of the ankle joint, subtalar joint, and the alignment of the calcaneus to the tibia. A study by Lamm and colleagues[26] showed a correlation between these frontal plane radiographic views and clinical assessment of the hindfoot. It is often difficult to obtain these images in the office. Having these performed by the radiology department ensures proper technique. These views have been helpful in preoperative planning for reconstruction of the AAFF.

AUTHORS' APPROACH TO SURGICAL MANAGEMENT OF FLEXIBLE AAFF

Patients with flexible stage II AAFF often have some degree of equinus deformity that requires lengthening of the posterior muscle group. This lengthening assists in

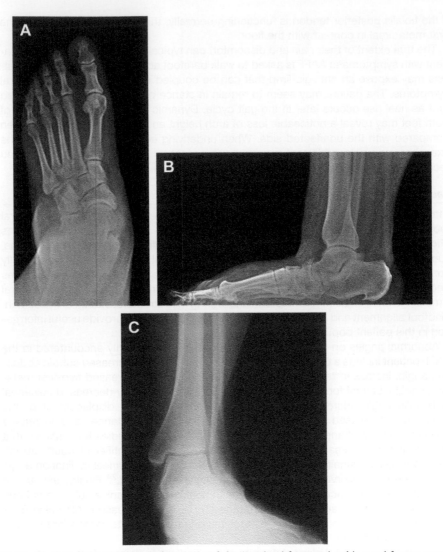

Fig. 3. (*A–C*) Standard radiographic views of the involved foot and ankle used for preoperative planning and patient education.

restoring calcaneal inclination and obtaining a plantigrade foot after osseous realignment. The authors perform a Strayer gastrocnemius soleus recession through a medial or posterior medial approach. However, there are times when the equinus deformity is severe enough to warrant an Achilles tendon lengthening. In these instances, a percutaneous triple hemisection or open frontal plane Z-lengthening is performed. However, the authors prefer the gastrocnemius soleus recession because of maintenance of muscle strength after the procedure.

Hindfoot valgus deformity associated with the nonfixed AAFF is addressed with a medializing calcaneal osteotomy (MCO) of the posterior calcaneus. It has been well established that the MCO is effective in reducing hindfoot valgus by redirecting the coronal vector of the Achilles tendon from eversion to inversion (**Fig. 4**).[6,27,28] The authors rarely use the MCO as an isolated procedure for stage II AAFF because, although

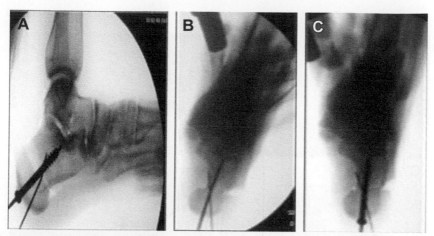

Fig. 4. (*A–C*) Use of the medializing calcaneal osteotomy to reduce heel valgus and realign the coronal vector of the Achilles tendon.

it has a direct effect on the subtalar joint, it has a much lesser effect on the midtarsal joint. In the senior author's experience (ARC, RD), most stage II deformities are too severe to be corrected by an isolated MCO. Vora and colleagues[29] evaluated the use of MCO in the correction of mild and severe flatfoot deformities. They concluded that severe deformities may require additional procedures to achieve correction of the deformity.[29] Lateral column lengthening (LCL) and MCO for reconstruction of AAFF were evaluated by Bolt and colleagues.[30] They found that those patients treated with isolated MCO were twice as likely to undergo reoperation because of inadequate realignment.[30] It is the authors' practice to use the MCO in conjunction with LCL.

The primary procedure for reconstruction of the flexible AAFF is LCL (Evans osteotomy) performed through an osteotomy of the anterior calcaneus (**Fig. 5**). Lengthening of the lateral column can also be performed through bone-block arthrodesis of the calcaneocuboid joint. This procedure has been abandoned by the authors due to the high rate of complications.[31–37] Cooper and colleagues[38] recommended the use of calcaneal-cuboid distraction arthrodesis to avoid joint arthrosis due to increases in calcaneal-cuboid joint pressure after Evans osteotomy. Momberger and colleagues[33] were able to refute these claims and show that lengthening of the lateral column does not increase calcaneal-cuboid joint pressures. In the senior author's experience, degenerative changes of this joint are rarely seen postoperative. LCL reduces the inversion demand on the PTT, reduces the Achilles force required to achieve heel rise, adducts and plantarflexes the midfoot relative to the hindfoot, and creates a "bowstringing" effect that may be responsible for restoration of the medial longitudinal arch.[39–41]

The authors have used allograft as their bone graft of choice for LCL through an anterior calcaneal osteotomy. Allograft has been shown to be acceptable and comparable to autograft for LCL.[42–45] A retrospective analysis of anterior calcaneal osteotomies using allograft bone performed by John and colleagues[44] demonstrated that allograft bone was safe and effective for LCL in AAFF reconstruction. The authors prefer iliac crest, or patellar wedge allograft, for its strong cortical structure in comparison to commercially available preformed wedges. These preformed wedges have much weaker cortical structure and often fracture during impaction into the osteotomy.

Fixation options for the anterior calcaneal osteotomy include no fixation, percutaneous Kirschner wire, small-diameter screw, and plate fixation. The authors prefer

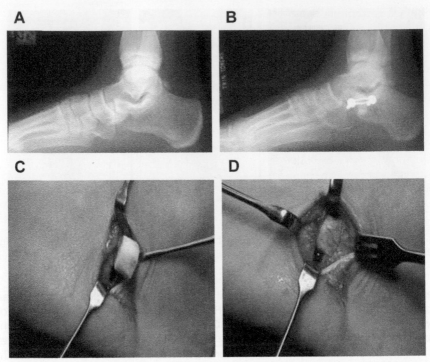

Fig. 5. (A–D) Lateral column lengthening with allograft bone graft creates adduction and plantarflexion of the midfoot on the hindfoot.

the use of one 4.0-mm cannulated screw inserted from the anterior process of the calcaneus proximal across the graft. These bone grafts are placed under a large amount of tension and displacement is unlikely; therefore, it is reasonable to believe that fixation is not required. Nonetheless, fixation secures the sagittal plane position of the bone graft and diminishes micro motion at the host-graft interface. The goal with fixation is to expedite bone graft incorporation and lessen the risk of nonunion. Plate fixation should be reserved as a secondary form of fixation for revision of nonunion or when bone cysts are present and being treated in the same setting. When plate fixation is used, patients often complain of symptoms secondary to peroneal tendon irritation, which has necessitated hardware removal in many of these cases. Dunn and Meyer[46] evaluated displacement of the anterior process of the calcaneus after LCL and concluded that fixation would inhibit late resorption of the dorsally displaced anterior process creating a potential source of pain or discomfort.

Lateral column pain is a noted complication after LCL and has been attributed to inappropriate graft size.[47–51] The authors commonly use an 8- to 10-mm graft. However, graft sizing can be an intraoperative challenge, and there are no guidelines to estimate the amount of lengthening necessary to reduce the deformity. A triangular or trapezoidal wedge may be used. Both shapes effectively lengthen the lateral column; however, a triangular wedge may decrease the amount of calcaneocuboid joint symptoms postoperatively. The authors have found that the magnitude of the deformity and suppleness of the soft tissues often influence the size of the graft that can be implanted. In cases of isolated LCL, one must often use a much larger graft. With the addition of MCO to LCL, one can control the amount of displacement required at both the osteotomy sites; this translates into the ability to use a smaller graft at the LCL site by increasing the amount of displacement at the MCO site. The authors routinely use a pin-based distracter to evaluate the amount of graft needed for deformity correction. The amount of correction can then be verified under fluoroscopy before insertion of the bone graft. Metal trial wedges can also be used to help ascertain graft size; however, the authors do not routinely use these (**Fig. 6**). The use of the trial wedges has been shown to decrease the incidence of postoperative lateral column pain and reduce eversion stiffness.[49]

The combination of LCL and MCO restores alignment in most cases of stage II AAFF. In the less severe cases, a joint-preserving medial cuneiform opening wedge osteotomy (MCOW or Cotton osteotomy) is performed to further stabilize the medial column and off-load the stress on the lateral column. In more severe cases, a medial column arthrodesis is required. This procedure can be either a naviculocuneiform

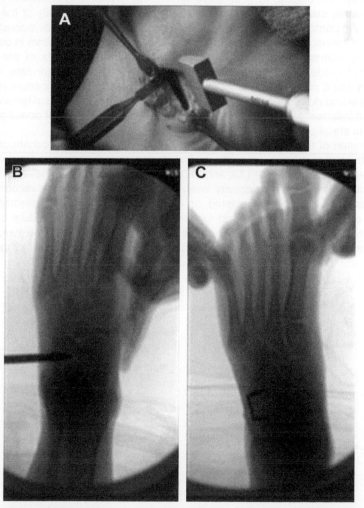

Fig. 6. (*A–C*) Use of trial wedges to evaluate graft size, deformity correction, and residual midfoot range of motion.

arthrodesis (NCA) or Miller procedure (naviculocuneiform and tarsometatarsal arthrodesis) used to address compensatory forefoot supinatus due to long-standing hindfoot valgus deformity (**Fig. 7**).

Forefoot supinatus, either nonfixed or fixed, that is left unaddressed results in failure of reconstruction of the AAFF. The NCA, or Miller procedure, is the authors' procedure of choice for fixed forefoot supinatus. Sagittal plane correction with NCA is accomplished by a combination of plantar rotation of the cuneiforms and/or wedge resection. Fixation is accomplished with crossed compression screws, compression plates, or a combination of plate and screw fixation. When performing the Miller procedure, the length of the medial column is maintained by placing femoral head allograft in the navicular-medial cuneiform arthrodesis site, as well as in the first metatarsal-medial cuneiform arthrodesis site. Fixation is accomplished with plate fixation that spans the medial column (**Fig. 8**).

In cases of supple, nonfixed, forefoot supinatus, the authors use the MCOW osteotomy (**Fig. 9**). This osteotomy is effective in reducing forefoot supinatus and restoring medial column stability.[47,52] Lutz and Myerson[52] confirmed the utility of the MCOW osteotomy in combination with other corrective procedures for flatfoot reconstruction. Hirose and Johnson[53] showed that this osteotomy is a powerful adjunct in correcting forefoot supinatus associated with flatfoot deformity. The benefits of the MCOW osteotomy include maintenance of first ray mobility, predictable union rate, ability to vary the amount of correction, and low complication rate.[53] The procedure is technically simple and does not require fixation because of the high amount of tension on the bone graft inserted. However, fixation with a small-diameter screw or dorsal plate can be used to stabilize the graft.

Stabilization of the medial column is a critical aspect of flatfoot reconstruction. Patients with medial column instability, or first ray instability, are at risk for developing lateral forefoot overload after LCL and MCO. These symptoms can develop after patients resume their preinjury activity level. Multiple researchers have recommended medial column arthrodesis, isolated or combined with hindfoot osteotomies, to improve overall foot alignment and function.[54,55] The authors' procedure of choice to impart stability to the medial column is the MCOW osteotomy. However, if there is evidence of joint arthrosis or global medial column instability (including a large

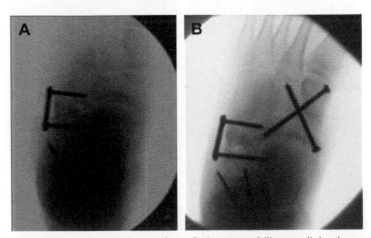

Fig. 7. (*A, B*) Addition of naviculocuneiform fusion to stabilize medial column, decrease forefoot supinatus, and reduce residual forefoot abduction.

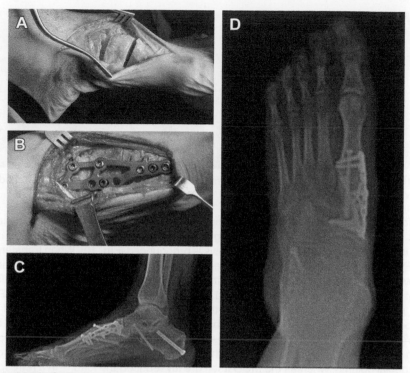

Fig. 8. (*A–D*) The Miller procedure reconstructs the medial column and imparts stability through arthrodesis of nonessential joints.

Meary angle), an NCA, first tarsometatarsal arthrodesis, or Miller procedure is performed. Arthrodesis of the medial column restores normal anatomy without fusing essential joints.[54]

Reconstruction of the soft-tissue structures is performed last and only if necessary. The PTT is explored and repaired if not severely degenerated. The degenerated

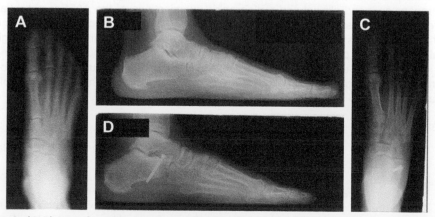

Fig. 9. (*A–D*) Use of medial cuneiform opening wedge osteotomy to reduce residual forefoot supinatus and restore medial column stability.

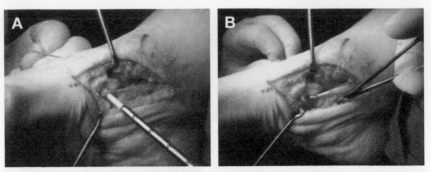

Fig. 10. (*A, B*) Transfer of flexor digitorum longus tendon to the navicular with biotenodesis screw fixation.

portions of the tendon are excised and the tendon is tubularized to maintain its excursion. Transfer of the flexor digitorum longus (FDL) is considered in cases in which the PTT is severely degenerated and tendinosis is pronounced (**Fig. 10**). When transferring the FDL tendon, the authors perform a tenodesis to the navicular with a biotenodesis screw. Osseous realignment is the most important factor relative to outcome. Realignment of the hindfoot supports the medial soft-tissue structures (spring ligament, PTT) and prevents further attenuation over the long term. The pathomechanics of the flatfoot contribute to the dysfunction of the PTT and spring ligament. Arangio and Salathe[56] conducted a biomechanical analysis of PTT dysfunction, MCO, and FDL transfer in AAFF. Their conclusions were that the FDL transfer did little to reduce the load on the medial column, whereas the MCO itself greatly reduced the load.[56] In a retrospective study of patients undergoing reconstruction for stage II AAFF, DiDomenico and colleagues[57] noted significant structural realignment without the use of FDL transfer. He concluded that the FDL transfer could be avoided without compromising the surgical outcome.

SUMMARY

Aggressive surgical management of stage II AAFF is important in preventing the progression of the deformity, adaptation of the osseous and soft-tissue structures, end-stage arthritis, and malalignment of the ankle. A thorough understanding of the pathoanatomy and clinical and radiographic examinations of the AAFF is essential. Preservation of essential joints through use of osteotomies, tendon transfers, and limited arthrodesis helps maintain motion and limit adjacent joint arthrosis. The surgical approach and procedure selection should be based on a thorough understanding of each patient's unique pathologic condition. Foot and ankle surgeons should be familiar with a set of procedures that address all pathologic components of the flexible stage II flatfoot.

REFERENCES

1. Johnson KA, Strom DE. Tibialis posterior tendon dysfunction. Clin Orthop Relat Res 1989;239:196–206.
2. Myerson MS. Adult acquired flatfoot deformity: treatment of dysfunction of the posterior tibial tendon. J Bone Joint Surg Am 1996;78:780–92.
3. Weinraub GM, Heilala MA. Adult flatfoot/posterior tibial tendon dysfunction: outcomes analysis of surgical treatment utilizing an algorithmic approach. J Foot Ankle Surg 2000;39:359–64.

4. Haddad SL, Myerson MS, Younger A, et al. Adult acquired flatfoot deformity. Foot Ankle Int 2011;32:95–111.
5. Bloome DM, Marymont JV, Varner KE. Variations of the insertion of the posterior tibial tendon: a cadaveric study. Foot Ankle Int 2003;24:780–3.
6. Giza G, Cush G, Schon LC. The flexible flatfoot in the adult. Foot Ankle Clin 2007;12:251–71.
7. Pinney SJ, Lin SS. Current concept review: acquired adult flatfoot deformity. Foot Ankle Int 2006;27:66–75.
8. Deland JT. The adult acquired flatfoot and spring ligament complex. Pathology and implications for treatment. Foot Ankle Clin 2001;6:129–35.
9. Brodsky JW. Preliminary gait analysis results after posterior tibial tendon reconstruction: a prospective study. Foot Ankle Int 2004;25:96–100.
10. Funk DA, Cass JR, Johnson KA. Acquired adult flat foot secondary to posterior tibial tendon pathology. J Bone Joint Surg Am 1986;68:95–102.
11. Pomeroy GC, Pike RH, Beals TC, et al. Acquired flatfoot in adults due to dysfunction of the posterior tibial tendon. J Bone Joint Surg Am 1999;81: 1173–82.
12. Geideman WM, Johnson JE. Posterior tibial tendon dysfunction. J Orthop Sports Phys Ther 2000;30:68–77.
13. Richie DH. Biomechanics and clinical analysis of the adult acquired flatfoot. Clin Podiatr Med Surg 2007;24:617–44.
14. Deland JT, de Asla RJ, Sung IH, et al. Posterior tibial tendon insufficiency: which ligaments are involved? Foot Ankle Int 2005;26:427–35.
15. Gazdag AR, Cracchiolo A 3rd. Rupture of the posterior tibial tendon. Evaluation of injury of the spring ligament and clinical assessment of tendon transfer and ligament repair. J Bone Joint Surg Am 1997;79:675–81.
16. Inman VT. Hallux valgus: a review of etiologic factors. Orthop Clin North Am 1974;5:59–66.
17. King DM, Toolan BC. Associated deformities and hypermobility in hallux valgus: an investigation with weightbearing radiographs. Foot Ankle Int 2004;25:251–5.
18. DiGiovanni CW, Langer P. The role of isolated gastrocnemius and combined Achilles contractures in the flatfoot. Foot Ankle Clin 2007;12:363–79.
19. DiGiovanni CW, Kuo R, Tejwani N, et al. Isolated gastrocnemius tightness. J Bone Joint Surg Am 2002;84:962–70.
20. Aronow MS. Triceps surae contractures associated with posterior tibial tendon dysfunction. Tech Orthop 2000;15:164–73.
21. Silverskiold N. Reduction of the uncrossed two-joint muscles of the leg to one-joint muscles in spastic conditions. Acta Chir Scand 1924;56:315–30.
22. Cass AD, Camasta CA. A review of tarsal coalition and pes planovalgus: clinical examination, diagnostic imaging, and surgical planning. J Foot Ankle Surg 2010;49:274–93.
23. Hintermann B, Gachter A. The first metatarsal rise sign: a simple sensitive sign of tibialis posterior tendon dysfunction. Foot Ankle Int 1996;17:236–41.
24. Younger AS, Sawatzky B, Dryden P. Radiographic assessment of adult flatfoot. Foot Ankle Int 2005;26:820–5.
25. Mendicino RW, Catanzariti AR, John S, et al. Long leg calcaneal axial and hindfoot alignment radiographic views for frontal plane assessment. J Am Podiatr Med Assoc 2008;98:75–8.
26. Lamm BM, Mendicino RW, Catanzariti AR, et al. Static rearfoot alignment: a comparison of clinical and radiographic measures. J Am Podiatr Med Assoc 2005;95:26–33.

27. Trnka HJ, Easley ME, Myerson MS. The role of calcaneal osteotomies for correction of adult flatfoot. Clin Orthop Relat Res 1999;365:50–64.
28. Den Hartog BD. Flexor digitorum longus transfer with medial displacement calcaneal osteotomy. Biomechanical rationale. Foot Ankle Clin 2001;6:67–76.
29. Vora AM, Tien TR, Parks BG, et al. Correction of moderate and severe acquired flexible flatfoot with medializing calcaneal osteotomy and flexor digitorum longus transfer. J Bone Joint Surg Am 2006;88:1726–34.
30. Bolt PM, Coy S, Toolan BC. A comparison of lateral column lengthening and medial translational osteotomy of the calcaneus for the reconstruction of adult acquired flatfoot. Foot Ankle Int 2007;28:1115–23.
31. Toolan BC, Sangeorzan BJ, Hansen ST Jr. Complex reconstruction for the treatment of dorsolateral peritalar subluxation of the foot. Early results after distraction arthrodesis of the calcaneocuboid joint in conjunction with stabilization of, and transfer of the flexor digitorum longus tendon to, the midfoot to treat acquired pes planovalgus in adults. J Bone Joint Surg Am 1999;81:1545–60.
32. Hintermann B, Valderrabano V, Kundert HP. Lengthening of the lateral column and reconstruction of the medial soft tissue for treatment of acquired flatfoot deformity associated with insufficiency of the posterior tibial tendon. Foot Ankle Int 1999;20:622–9.
33. Momberger N, Morgan JM, Bachus KN, et al. Calcaneocuboid joint pressure after lateral column lengthening in a cadaveric planovalgus deformity model. Foot Ankle Int 2000;21:730–5.
34. Moseir-LaClair S, Pomeroy G, Manoli A 2nd. Intermediate follow-up on the double osteotomy and tendon transfer procedure for stage II posterior tibial tendon insufficiency. Foot Ankle Int 2001;22:283–91.
35. Conti SF, Wong YS. Osteolysis of structural autograft after calcaneocuboid distraction arthrodesis for stage II posterior tibial tendon dysfunction. Foot Ankle Int 2002;23:521–9.
36. Thomas RL, Wells BC, Garrison RL, et al. Preliminary results comparing two methods of lateral column lengthening. Foot Ankle Int 2001;22:107–19.
37. Haeseker GA, Mureau MA, Faber F. Lateral column lengthening for acquired adult flatfoot deformity caused by posterior tibial tendon dysfunction stage II. J Foot Ankle Surg 2010;49:380–4.
38. Cooper PS, Nowak MD, Shaer J. Calcaneocuboid joint pressures with lateral column lengthening (Evans) procedure. Foot Ankle Int 1997;18:199–205.
39. Sung IL, Lee S, Otis JC, et al. Posterior tibial tendon force requirements in early heel rise after calcaneal osteotomies. Foot Ankle Int 2002;23:842–9.
40. Mosca VS. Calcaneal lengthening for valgus deformity of the hindfoot. Results in children who had severe, symptomatic flatfoot and skewfoot. J Bone Joint Surg Am 1995;77:500–12.
41. Dumontier TA, Falicov A, Mosca V, et al. Calcaneal lengthening: investigation of deformity correction in a cadaveric flatfoot model. Foot Ankle Int 2005;26:166–70.
42. Mahan KT, Hillstrom HJ. Bone grafting in foot and ankle surgery. A review of 300 cases. J Am Podiatr Med Assoc 1998;88:109–18.
43. Dolan CM, Henning JA, Anderson JG, et al. Randomized prospective study comparing tri-cortical iliac crest autograft to allograft in the lateral column lengthening component for operative correction of adult acquired flatfoot deformity. Foot Ankle Int 2007;28:8–12.
44. John S, Child BJ, Hix J, et al. A retrospective analysis of anterior calcaneal osteotomy with allogenic bone graft. J Foot Ankle Surg 2010;49:375–9.

45. Grier KM, Walling AK. The use of tricortical autograft versus allograft in lateral column lengthening for adult acquired flatfoot deformity. Foot Ankle Int 2010; 31:760–9.
46. Dunn SP, Meyer J. Displacement of the anterior process of the calcaneus after evans calcaneal osteotomy. J Foot Ankle Surg 2011;50:402–6.
47. Benthien RA, Parks BG, Guyton GP, et al. Lateral column lengthening, flexor digitorum longus tendon transfer, and opening wedge medial cuneiform osteotomy for flexible flatfoot: a biomechanical study. Foot Ankle Int 2007;28:70–7.
48. Oh I, Williams BR, Ellis SJ, et al. Reconstruction of the symptomatic idiopathic flatfoot in adolescents and young adults. Foot Ankle Int 2011;32:225–32.
49. Ellis SJ, Williams BR, Garg R, et al. Incidence of plantar lateral foot pain before and after the use of trial metal wedges in lateral column lengthening. Foot Ankle Int 2011;32:665–73.
50. Ellis SJ, Yu JC, Johnson AH, et al. Plantar pressures in patients with and without lateral foot pain after lateral column lengthening. J Bone Joint Surg Am 2010;92: 81–91.
51. Deland JT, Page A, Sung IH, et al. Posterior tibial tendon insufficiency results at different stages. HSS J 2006;2:157–60.
52. Lutz M, Myerson M. Radiographic analysis of an opening wedge osteotomy of the medial cuneiform. Foot Ankle Int 2011;32:278–87.
53. Hirose CB, Johnson JE. Plantarflexion opening wedge medial cuneiform osteotomy for correction of fixed forefoot varus associated with flatfoot deformity. Foot Ankle Int 2004;25:568–74.
54. Greisberg J, Assal M, Hansen ST. Isolated medial column stabilization improves alignment in adult-acquired flatfoot. Clin Orthop Relat Res 2005;435:197–202.
55. Jordan TH, Rush SM, Hamilton GA, et al. Radiographic outcomes of adult acquired flatfoot corrected by medial column arthrodesis with or without medializing calcaneal osteotomy. J Foot Ankle Surg 2011;50:176–81.
56. Arangio GA, Salathe EP. A biomechanical analysis of posterior tibial tendon dysfunction, medial displacement calcaneal osteotomy and flexor digitorum longus transfer in adult acquired flat foot. Clin Biomech 2009;24:385–90.
57. DiDomenico L, Stein DY, Wargo-Dorsey M. Treatment of posterior tibial tendon dysfunction with flexor digitorum tendon transfer: a retrospective study of 34 patients. J Foot Ankle Surg 2011;50:293–8.

Surgical Management of Stage 2 Adult Acquired Flatfoot

Jared M. Maker, DPM, AACFAS[a],*, James M. Cottom, DPM, FACFAS[b]

KEYWORDS

- Adult acquired flatfoot deformity • Stage 2 flatfoot deformity
- Posterior tibial tendon dysfunction • Flexor digitorum longus tendon transfer
- Calcaneal osteotomy

KEY POINTS

- Adult acquired flatfoot deformity is a progressive disorder with multiple symptoms and degrees of deformity.
- Stage II adult acquired flatfoot can be divided into stage IIA and IIB based on severity of deformity.
- Surgical procedures should be chosen based on severity as well as location of the flatfoot deformity.
- Care must be taken not to overcorrect the flatfoot deformity so as to decrease the possibility of lateral column overload as well as stiffness.

INTRODUCTION

Adult acquired flatfoot deformity (AAFD) is a progressive as well as intricate disorder with multiple symptoms and numerous degrees of deformity.[1,2] Johnson and Strom[3] originally described 3 stages of AAFD that are practical when determining treatment options.[1] Stage I patients complain of aching along the medial ankle without having secondary deformity. In stage II, pain increases in severity and distribution. The posterior tibial tendon (PTT) is elongated with secondary forefoot abduction as well as hindfoot valgus.[3] Stage II has been further branched into stages IIa and IIb.[4–6] Stage IIa has minimal abduction deformity through the midfoot with anterior-posterior (AP) radiographs revealing less than 30% talar head uncoverage. Patients with stage IIb reveal increased deformity on examination with AP radiographs revealing greater than 30% talar head uncoverage.[4,5] Stage III has complete disruption of the PTT, with the patient having a fixed hindfoot valgus position along with secondary degenerative changes in

[a] Foot and Ankle Surgical Fellowship, Coastal Orthopedics and Sports Medicine, 6015 Pointe West Boulevard, Bradenton, FL 34209, USA; [b] Coastal Orthopedics and Sports Medicine, 6015 Pointe West Boulevard, Bradenton, FL 34209, USA
* Corresponding author.
E-mail address: jmaker@coastalorthopedics.com

Clin Podiatr Med Surg 31 (2014) 381–389
http://dx.doi.org/10.1016/j.cpm.2014.03.002
0891-8422/14/$ – see front matter © 2014 Elsevier Inc. All rights reserved.

the tritarsal complex.[3] Myerson[7] later described stage IV AAFD as valgus angulation of the talus along with degenerative changes within the ankle joint.

PATIENT PHYSICAL EXAMINATION

When performing a physical examination in the AAFD, the patient must be assessed in the relaxed stance position. When examining in the standing position, the forefoot may appear abducted in relationship to the rearfoot, causing the medial border to have a bulging and convex appearance with the lateral border shortened and concave.[8] Forefoot abduction also is assessed from behind the patient with the "too many toes" sign. As an increase in severity of the deformity occurs, an increase in the number of toes laterally will be visualized.[8,9] Commonly, a valgus deformity of the heel will be visualized as well.[10]

Following the stance examination, the reducibility of the deformity should be assessed. Single heel rise test is important to the examination when determining the function of the PTT with respect to stability of the arch. With a nonfunctioning PTT, the sagittal plane will reveal plantar flexion of the rearfoot on the forefoot. Minimal to no elevation of the heel will be visualized.[10] When a patient is able to do a single heel rise, close examination of whether the heel shifts into varus must be assessed. The single heel rise test is positive if either the patient cannot elevate the heel off the ground or the heel does not shift into varus, staying in valgus during heel lift.[4] Assessment of the reducibility of heel valgus can also be done with the double heel rise test.[2]

Range of motion (ROM) should be assessed at the ankle joint with the knee flexed and extended to determine if there is a gastrocnemius-soleus equinus or gastrocnemius equinus deformity. ROM should also be assessed at the subtalar joint.[11] If the subtalar joint is unable to be reduced, reconstructive options may be inhibited.[1,7,12] Assessment of PTT may reveal discomfort or fullness on palpation.[11] Finally, PTT muscle strength of the affected limb should be assessed in relation to the contralateral side.[10]

IMAGING

With stage II AAFD, radiographic analysis should be performed to assess the severity of the deformity. Typically, AP, lateral, medial oblique, ankle, and hindfoot alignment views are routinely done. Measurements on the AP view consist of talar first metatarsal angle, calcaneocuboid abduction angle, as well as talar head coverage when evaluating the amount of pronation and forefoot abduction. Measurements on the lateral view include talar first metatarsal angle and calcaneal inclination angle.[2] The hindfoot alignment view allows the assessment of the frontal plane alignment of the calcaneus in relation to the tibia (**Figs. 1** and **2**).[2,13,14]

When evaluating the PTT, magnetic resonance imaging (MRI) will detect sheath inflammation, soft tissue resolution, and the current anatomic state of the tendon.[15,16] Wacker and colleagues[17] compared the muscle belly of the PTT and FDL tendon with MRI in patients with AAFD. Patients with complete rupture of the PTT revealed fatty infiltration within the muscle belly, therefore being nonfunctional. PTT without complete rupture showed 10.7% atrophy of the muscle belly and 17.2% hypertrophy of the FDL muscle belly. This study demonstrates the use of MRI with regards to surgical planning. With a complete rupture, augmenting the transferred FDL tendon to the PTT likely will not contribute much function.[16]

CONSERVATIVE THERAPY

Conservative therapy consists of a multitude of modalities including immobilization, anti-inflammatories, physical therapy, and bracing. A study by Nielsen and colleagues[18]

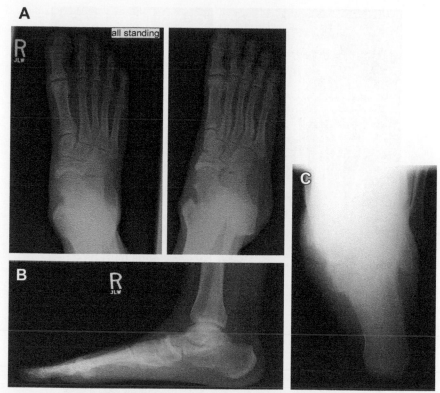

Fig. 1. AP (*A*), lateral (*B*), and axial-calcaneal (*C*) of a patient with stage IIA AAFD. Patient has less than 30% talar head uncoverage (*A*), along with decreased calcaneal inclination angle (*B*), and increased calcaneal valgus deformity (*C*).

using these modalities revealed symptoms were alleviated in 87.5% of patients preventing surgical intervention. Another study using nonoperative therapy by Alvarez and colleagues[19] consisting of short articulated ankle-foot orthosis, foot orthosis, and physical therapy showed an 89% satisfaction rate. These studies show that conservative therapy does have a benefit at alleviating symptoms and improving patient's satisfaction. When these fail to improve symptoms, surgical intervention is then performed.

STAGE II SURGICAL TECHNIQUE

A contracted gastrocnemius-soleus complex has been shown to increase forefoot and midfoot pressures, in turn causing increased stress along the medial arch.[20–23] Before correcting deformity in the foot, the senior author addresses the equinus contracture. With a gastrocnemius equinus, a gastrocnemius recession is performed, as described by Strayer.[24] Repair of the deep fascia is included in the closure following an adequate recession. When the equinus deformity is caused by both the gastrocnemius and the soleus muscles, a percutaneous tendo-achilles lengthening procedure is then used. Correcting the soft tissue contracture in this area should be considered to place the calcaneus successfully in the rectus position with flatfoot reconstruction. A continued contracture can lead to an undercorrected deformity.[25]

After addressing the equinus contracture, the procedures chosen for correction of the flatfoot deformity are determined based on the amount along with location of

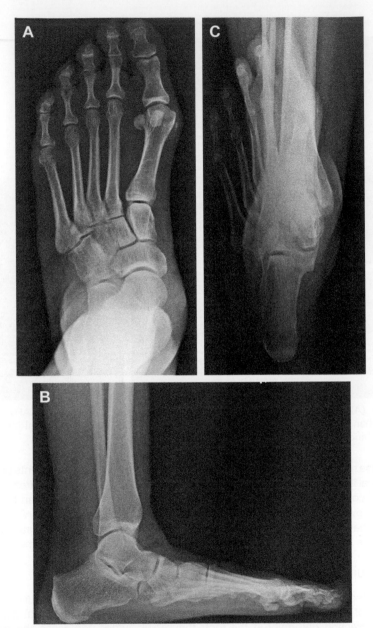

Fig. 2. AP (*A*), lateral (*B*), axial-calcaneal (*C*) of patient with stage IIB AAFD. Note the talar head uncoverage of greater than 30% (*A*), decrease in the calcaneal inclination angle, and increase in the talar-first metatarsal angle (*B*), and calcaneal valgus (*C*).

deformity.[4] With a mild, flexible deformity (stage IIA), successful reconstruction can be achieved with a medial calcaneal displacement osteotomy (MCDO) along with a flexor digitorum longus (FDL) tendon transfer. The MCDO has been studied and shown to correct heel valgus and alleviate the PTT and medial ligaments from excessive strain, therefore improving function and alignment, as well as relieving pain. These results make this the reconstructive procedure of choice for flatfoot deformity (**Fig. 3**).[26–32]

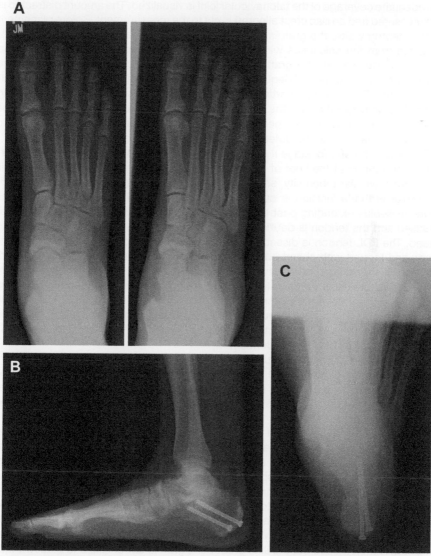

Fig. 3. AP (*A*), lateral (*B*), and axial-calcaneal (*C*) of the same patient from **Fig. 1** with stage IIA AAFD following gastrocnemius recession, FDL tendon transfer, and MCDO. Patient has an improved calcaneal inclination angle and talar-first metatarsal angle (*B*) as well as a rectus calcaneus on the axial calcaneal view (*C*).

When the patient presents with a more severe deformity (stage IIB), having increased talar head uncoverage and midfoot abduction, a double calcaneal osteotomy will be performed along with the FDL tendon transfer. Lateral column lengthening is a powerful procedure, increasing the arch, and correcting the abducted talonavicular joint.[33] The senior author makes the anterior calcaneal osteotomy before the MCDO. This osteotomy site is made 13 mm from the calcaneocuboid joint to prevent damage to the anterior and middle facets of the calcaneus.[34] Pins are placed proximal and distal to the osteotomy site. With a distractor, under fluoroscopy, the osteotomy site is mobilized until adequate coverage of the talonavicular joint is visualized. The amount distracted is then measured and an iliac crest allograft is cut to the measurement. Before placement in the osteotomy site, the graft is supersaturated with bone marrow aspirate (BMA) harvested from the calcaneus with the technique described by Schweinberger and Roukis.[35] Once placed, the graft is secured with a single cannulated screw. The MCDO is then performed. Adequate displacement is confirmed with a calcaneal-axial view and fixated with 2 partially threaded cannulated screws. When performing a lateral column lengthening, the surgeon should be careful not to overcorrect the deformity. Lateral column lengthening increases pressures of the lateral column and decreases eversion, with the potential of causing considerable stiffness.[4,36,37]

FDL tendon transfer for stage II AAFD has been performed with a long incision, harvesting the tendon at the knot of Henry. The tendon was then routed through a drill hole at the navicular tuberosity, securing the tendon by suturing to the periosteum.[38] The senior author's incision is curvilinear and placed at the inferior aspect of the medial malleolus extending past the navicular tuberosity 1.5–2 cm. The PTT sheath is incised and the tendon is debrided. The FDL tendon sheath is then identified and incised. The FDL tendon is dissected out distally, harvested proximal to the knot of Henry, and tagged with absorbable suture, and the diameter is appropriately sized. A drill hole is then placed in the navicular tuberosity dorsal to plantar under direct fluoroscopic guidance with care not to fracture through medially. The tendon is secured under proper tension with a biotenodesis screw. If the PTT is intact, the FDL tendon is sutured to the PTT before closure. A study by Wukich and colleagues[39] achieved patient satisfaction without clinical failure in 92% of patients using a biotenodesis screw for fixation of the FDL tendon.

Failure to address forefoot varus deformity may lead to a failed flatfoot surgery.[25] First described by Cotton,[40] the plantar flexion opening wedge osteotomy of the medial cuneiform is a common procedure to improve the declination of the first ray and restore a normal talo-first metatarsal relationship.[16] A study by Hirose and Johnson[41] specifically looked at the Cotton osteotomy. The union rate was 100% with patients having no to mild pain with ambulation. Radiographs revealed an improved talus-first metatarsal angle and medial cuneiform-to-floor height. They also noted the ability to vary the amount of correction through adjusting the wedge width and taper. When performing this procedure, the senior author exposes medial cuneiform through a dorsal incision and identifies the osteomy site under fluoroscopy. The osteotomy is made dorsal-to-plantar and a distractor is placed spanning the osteotomy site. The area is distracted until the varus deformity is reduced clinically with the first metatarsal head in line with the lesser metatarsal heads. The area distracted is then measured; the iliac crest bone graft is cut to size and placed within the gap. Before placement of the graft, it is supersaturated with BMA harvested from the calcaneus as discussed with lateral column lengthening (**Fig. 4**).

POSTOPERATIVE COURSE

Immediately following the procedure, the senior author places the patient in a posterior splint for 14 days. At the first postoperative visit, the splint is removed and the patient is then placed in a below-the-knee non-weight-bearing cast for 1 week. At the 3-week mark, sutures and staples are removed and the patient is placed in a below-the-knee walking cast at 100% weight-bearing for 2 weeks. At 5 weeks, the patient is transitioned into a pneumatic fracture boot and physical therapy is initiated. Return to regular shoe gear occurs between 6 and 7 weeks, along with a temporary ankle brace for continued protection of the repair.

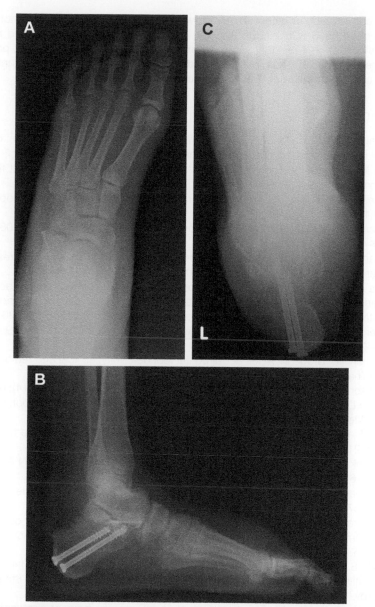

Fig. 4. AP (*A*), lateral (*B*), and axial-calcaneal (*C*) of the same patient from **Fig. 2** with stage IIB AAFD following a gastrocnemius recession, FDL tendon transfer, lateral calcaneal lengthening osteotomy, and MCDO. Patient had improved calcaneal inclination angle following the double calcaneal osteotomy as well as a parallel talar-first metatarsal angle (*B*). Medial column stabilization was not needed in this patient.

SUMMARY

AAFD is a progressive disorder that if not addressed can lead to a debilitating deformity. When conservative measures fail to relieve symptoms, surgical intervention should be performed. In stage IIA AAFD, patients do relatively well with FDL tendon transfer and MCDO. In stage IIB AAFD, where the deformity is more pronounced, patients often need FDL tendon transfer, double calcaneal osteotomy, and medial column stabilization if residual varus deformity is present. In stage II AAFD, patients should be evaluated and surgically repaired in a methodical manner so as to not over-correct, causing possible stiffness and lateral column overload.

REFERENCES

1. Catanzariti AR, Lee MS, Mendicino RW. Posterior calcaneal displacement osteotomy for adult acquired flatfoot deformity. J Foot Ankle Surg 2000;39(1):2–14.
2. Lee MS, Vanore JV, Thomas JL, et al. Diagnosis and treatment of adult flatfoot. J Foot Ankle Surg 2005;44(2):78–113.
3. Johnson KA, Strom DE. Tibialis posterior tendon dysfunction. Clin Orthop 1989; 239:196–206.
4. Deland JT. Adult acquired flatfoot deformity. J Am Acad Orthop Surg 2008;16(7): 399–406.
5. Deland JT, Page A, Sung IH, et al. Posterior tibial tendon insufficiency results at different stages. HSS J 2006;2:157–60.
6. Vora AM, Tien TR, Parks BG, et al. Correction of moderate and severe acquired flexible flatfoot with medializing calcaneal displacement osteotomy and flexor digitorum longus tendon transfer. J Bone Joint Surg Am 2006;88(8):1726–34.
7. Myerson MS. Adult acquired flatfoot deformity. J Bone Joint Surg Am 1996;78(5): 780–92.
8. Meehan RE, Brage M. Adult acquired flat foot deformity: clinical and radiographic examination. Foot Ankle Clin 2003;8(4):431–52.
9. Johnson KA. Tibialis posterior tendon rupture. Clin Orthop 1983;177(4):140–7.
10. Richie DH. Biomechanics and clinical analysis of adult acquired flatfoot. Clin Podiatr Med Surg 2007;24(4):617–44.
11. Giza E, Cush G, Shon LC. The flexible flatfoot in the adult. Foot Ankle Clin 2007; 12(2):215–394.
12. Slovenkae MP. Clinical and radiographic evaluation. Foot Ankle Clin N Am 1997; 2:241 60.
13. Saltzman CL, El-Khoury GY. The hindfoot alignment view. Foot Ankle Int 1995; 16(9):572–6.
14. Catanzariti AR, Mendicino RW, King GL, et al. Double calcaneal osteotomy: realignment considerations in eight patients. J Am Podiatr Med Assoc 2005; 95(1):53–9.
15. Woll TS. Posterior tibial tendon dysfunction. West J Med 1993;159(4):485–6.
16. Coughlin MJ, Mann RA, Saltzman CL. Surgery of the foot and ankle. 8th edition. Mosby, Inc; 2007. p. 1007–85.
17. Wacker JT, Calder JD, Engstrom CM, et al. MR morphometry of posterior tibialis muscle in adult acquired flatfoot. Foot Ankle Int 2003;24(4):354–7.
18. Nielsen MD, Dodson EE, Shadrick DL, et al. Nonoperative care for the treatment of adult-acquired flatfoot deformity. J Foot Ankle Surg 2011;50(3):311–4.
19. Alvarez RG, Marini A, Schmitt C, et al. Stage I and II posterior tibial tendon dysfunction treated by a structured non-operative management protocol: an orthosis and exercise program. Foot Ankle Int 2010;27(1):2–8.
20. Meszaros A, Caudell G. The surgical management of equinus in the adult acquired flatfoot. Clin Podiatr Med Surg 2007;24(4):667–85.
21. Jones RL. The human foot. An experimental study of its mechanics and the role of its muscles and ligaments in the support of the arch. Am J Anat 1941;68:1–38.

22. Ward ED, Phillips RD, Patterson PE, et al. The effects of extrinsic muscle forces on the forefoot-to-rearfoot loading relationship in vitro. J Am Podiatr Med Assoc 1998;88:471–82.
23. Aronow MS, Diaz-Doran V, Sullivan RJ, et al. The effect of triceps surae contracture force on plantar foot pressure distribution. Foot Ankle Int 2006;27(1):43–52.
24. Strayer LM. Recession of the gastrocnemius: an operation to relieve spastic contracture of the calf muscle. J Bone Joint Surg Am 1950;32(3):671–6.
25. Lee MS, Maker JM. Revision of failed flatfoot surgery. Clin Podiatr Med Surg 2009; 26(1):47–58.
26. Niki H, Hirano T, Okada H, et al. Outcome of medial displacement calcaneal osteotomy for correction of adult-acquired flatfoot. Foot Ankle Int 2012;33(11): 940–6.
27. Guyton GP, Jeng C, Krieger LE, et al. Flexor digitorum longus transfer and medial displacement calcaneal osteotomy for posterior tibial tendon dysfunction: a middle-term clinical follow-up. Foot Ankle Int 2001;22(8):627–32.
28. Myerson MS, Badekas A, Schon LC. Treatment of stage II posterior tibial tendon deficiency with flexor digitorum longus tendon transfer and calcaneal osteotomy. Foot Ankle Int 2004;25(7):445–50.
29. Myerson MS, Corrigan J, Thompson F, et al. Tendon transfer combined with calcaneal osteotomy for treatment of posterior tibial tendon insufficiency: a radiological investigation. Foot Ankle Int 1995;16:712–8.
30. Sammarco GJ, Hockenbury RT. Treatment of stage II posterior tibial tendon dysfunction with flexor hallucis longus tendon transfer and medial displacement calcaneal osteotomy. Foot Ankle Int 2001;22(4):305–12.
31. Wacker JT, Hennessy MS, Saxby TS. Calcaneal osteotomy and transfer of the tendon of flexor digitorum longus for stage-II dysfunction of tibialis posterior. Three to five year results. J Bone Joint Surg Br 2002;84(1):54–8.
32. Otis JC, Deland JT, Kenneally S, et al. Medial arch strain after medial displacement calcaneal osteotomy: an in vitro study. Foot Ankle Int 1999;20(4):222–6.
33. DuMontier TA, Falicov A, Mosca V, et al. Calcaneal lengthening: investigation of deformity correction in a cadaver flatfoot model. Foot Ankle Int 2005;26(2):166–70.
34. Hyer CF, Lee T, Block AJ, et al. Evaluation of the anterior and middle talocalcaneal articular facets and the Evans osteotomy. J Foot Ankle Surg 2002;41(6):389–93.
35. Schweinberger MH, Roukis TS. Percutaneous autologous bone marrow harvest from the calcaneus and proximal tibia: surgical technique. J Foot Ankle Surg 2007;46(5):411–4.
36. Tien TR, Parks BG, Guyton GP. Plantar pressures in the forefoot after lateral column lengthening: a cadaver study comparing the Evans osteotomy and calcaneocuboid fusion. Foot Ankle Int 2005;26(7):520–5.
37. Thomas RL, Wells BC, Garrison RL, et al. Preliminary results comparing two methods of lateral column lengthening. Foot Ankle Int 2001;22(2):107–19.
38. Mann RA, Coughlin MJ. Surgery of the foot and ankle. 7th edition. Mosby, Inc; 1999. p. 200–10.
39. Wukich DK, Bora R, Lowery NJ, et al. Biotenodesis screw for fixation of FDL transfer in the treatment of adult acquired flatfoot deformity. Foot Ankle Int 2008;29(7): 730–4.
40. Cotton FJ. Foot statics and surgery. N Engl J Med 1936;214:353–62.
41. Hirose CB, Johnson JE. Plantar flexion opening wedge medial cuneiform osteotomy for correction of fixed forefoot varus associated with flatfoot deformity. Foot Ankle Int 2004;25(8):568–74.

Addressing Stage II Posterior Tibial Tendon Dysfunction

Biomechanically Repairing the Osseous Structures Without the Need of Performing the Flexor Digitorum Longus Transfer

Lawrence A. DiDomenico, DPM[a,b,c,]*, Zachary M. Thomas, DPM[c], Ramy Fahim, DPM, AACFAS[a]

KEYWORDS

- Posterior tibial tendon dysfunction • Adult acquired flatfoot deformity
- Flexor digitorum longus • Calcaneal slide osteotomy

KEY POINTS

- A double calcaneal osteotomy, a gastrocnemius recession and stabilization of the medial column provides satisfactory correction, stability, and realignment of the foot.
- The use of the flexor digitorum longus transfer, can be avoided without compromising the outcome when surgically treating posterior tibial tendon dysfunction.

INTRODUCTION

Adult acquired flatfoot deformity is characterized by collapse of the medial longitudinal arch and loss of the mechanical advantage of the posterior-medial soft-tissue structures, including the posterior tibial tendon. Key[1] initially described a chronic partial rupture of the posterior tibial tendon in 1953.

Further literature confirmed an association with this abnormality and, in fact, "dysfunction" of this posterior tibial tendon with adult acquired flatfoot deformity. The clinical presentation of adult flatfoot can range from a flexible deformity with normal joint integrity to a rigid, arthritic flat foot. Conservative and surgical management of flatfoot deformity has been reviewed extensively in the literature, but debate still exists regarding the surgical management of stage II deformities, especially in the presence of medial column instability. Historically triple arthrodesis was a common surgical approach; however, the increased incidence and awareness of posterior tibial

[a] Ankle & Foot Care Centers, 8175 Market Street, Youngstown, OH 44512, USA; [b] St. Elizabeth Hospital, Youngstown, Ohio; [c] Heritage Valley Hospital, Beaver, Pennsylvania, USA
* Corresponding author.
E-mail address: ld5353@aol.com

Clin Podiatr Med Surg 31 (2014) 391–404
http://dx.doi.org/10.1016/j.cpm.2014.03.008
0891-8422/14/$ – see front matter © 2014 Elsevier Inc. All rights reserved.

podiatric.theclinics.com

tendon dysfunction has stimulated a trend toward surgical interventions that involve joint preservation techniques.[2,3]

The purpose of this article is to review and discuss various surgical options for the correction of stage II flatfoot reconstructive procedures. The authors discuss their opinion that is not always necessary to transfer the flexor digitorum longus tendon to provide relief and stability in this patient population. The article focuses on the anatomy, diagnosis, and current treatments of flexible flatfoot deformity (**Fig. 1**).

FUNCTIONAL ANATOMY

The tibialis posterior arises from the posterior aspect of the tibia and is part of the deep posterior compartment. The tendon divides in the proximity to the navicular tuberosity into 3 slips: the anterior, middle, and posterior. The anterior slip is the largest of these, and also is the slip considered to be the continuation of the posterior tibial tendon proper. This slip inserts on to the navicular tuberosity, first cuneiform-navicular joint, and inferior first cuneiform. The middle tendon slip fans out like multiple tentacles that travel deep into the plantar vault of the foot inserting on the second and third cuneiform, lateral second metatarsal base, medial and lateral third metatarsal base, medial fourth metatarsal base, and cuboid. Occasionally there is a slip to the fifth metatarsal base. At the level of the midfoot this portion of tendon gives origin to the flexor hallucis brevis. The tendon also crosses deep to the peroneus longus and, in some instances, directly interacts with this tendon by tendinous attachment. The posterior component of the tibialis posterior travels lateral and posterior to insert on the sustentaculum tali.[4] Ultrasonographic imaging of the tibialis posterior shows a mean width of 9.72 to 11.12 mm, thickness of 3.42 to 3.64 mm, and cross-sectional area of 2.66 to 3.07 mm^2 based on 3 observers. Magnetic resonance imaging (MRI) shows measurements of 10.65 to 11.11 mm width, thickness of 3.95 to 4.18 mm, and cross-sectional area of 3.17 to 4.06 mm^2.[5]

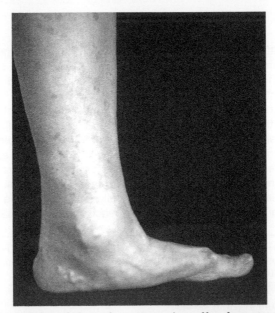

Fig. 1. Medial aspect of the left foot of a patient who suffers from stage II posterior tibial tendon dysfunction.

The flexor digitorum longus originates from the posterior tibia and interosseous membrane. The tendon courses under the sustentaculum tali as part of the deep posterior compartment. The tendon of the flexor digitorum longus traverses plantar to the flexor hallucis longus and travels anteriorly and laterally before it splits in to 4 slips, each inserting on their respective lesser digital distal phalanx. The tendon of the flexor digitorum longus also gives origin to the quadratus plantae.[4] Ultrasonographic measurements of the flexor digitorum longus show a mean cross-sectional area of 1.59 to 176 mm^2.[6]

The course of the posterior tibial tendon runs slightly superior to the flexor digitorum longus. The flexor digitorum longus runs in a more axial fashion than the posterior tibial tendon. The higher angle of descent of the posterior tibial tendon places it in the ideal location for its strap-like, arch-supporting function.

When transferring the flexor digitorum longus to the posterior tibial tendon insertion, the flexor digitorum longus cannot recreate the trajectory of the posterior tibial tendon. Moreover, when transferring the flexor digitorum longus into the navicular or medial cuneiform, the tentacle-like insertions of the posterior tibial tendon are sacrificed.

In addition the spring ligament, the deltoid ligament complex, and the articular relationship of the talonavicular and subtalar joints can be affected in the presence of posterior tibial tendon dysfunction.

The vascularity of the posterior tibial tendon originates from branches of the posterior tibial artery. Superior to the medial malleolus, the posterior tibial tendon has vessels in the synovial sheath, which come from muscle tissue. Distally the insertion receives its blood supply from the periosteal tissue. In between is a zone of hypovascularity, which often corresponds to the site of the diseased tendon.[7]

PATHOLOGY

Biomechanical imbalance can lead to chronic microtrauma in the posterior tibial tendon. In addition, advanced age lessens tendon elasticity because of changes in collagen structure that create tendon weakness.[8] Poor blood supply may stimulate this disease process and may preclude healing of the tendon, leading to a chronic inflammatory state that creates tenosynovitis and tendinosis. Deland and colleagues[9] demonstrated that medial calcaneonavicular ligaments and the interosseous ligament are often implicated in posterior tibial tendon dysfunction. Other causes include medical conditions such as ligamentous laxity and trauma to the posterior tibial tendon. More common are biomechanical conditions associated with posterior tibial dysfunction. This patient population typically presents with an equinus contracture, a medial column instability that can lead to a forefoot varus and a hindfoot valgus.

CLASSIFICATION

Johnson and Strom[10] described 3 stages of posterior tibial tendon dysfunction, with Myerson and Bluman[11] describing a fourth stage.

Stage I is described as painful tenosynovitis of the posterior tibial tendon. The patient is able to perform a single-limb heel rise. The hindfoot is supple. In this stage, a period of immobilization in a walking cast or walking boot followed by either ankle-foot orthosis or an orthotic can often manage this condition successfully.

Stage II is characterized by an elongated posterior tibial tendon, medial pain, and a mobile hindfoot valgus that corrects to neutral on heel rise. A single-limb heel-rise test shows marked weakness. There is a positive "too many toes" sign. Stage II can also be subdivided into IIA (<30% uncovering of talar head), IIB (>30% uncovering of talar head), and IIC, which is stage II posterior tibial tendon dysfunction with associated forefoot varus (**Fig. 2**).

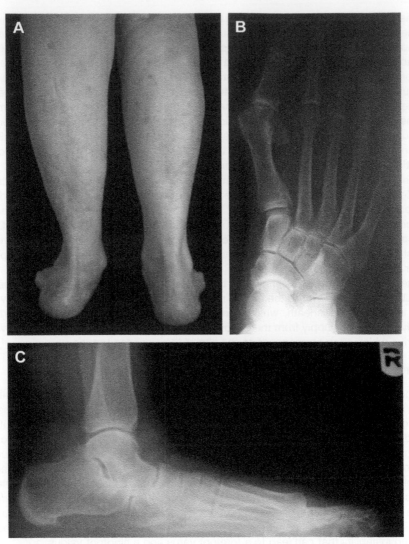

Fig. 2. (*A*) A patient diagnosed with stage II posterior tibial tendon dysfunction. Note the "too many toes" sign, calcaneal valgus malalignment, posterior-medial bulge, and forefoot abduction of the left foot. (*B*) Anteroposterior (AP) radiograph of a patient who suffers from posterior tibial tendon dysfunction. Note the malalignment and malrotation of the midtarsal joint. (*C*) Lateral radiograph showing the malalignment of the hindfoot and mid-foot. Note the elevated first metatarsal demonstrating instability of first tarsometatarsal.

Stage III is rigid hindfoot valgus that does not correct on double-limb heel rise. The patient may not be able to perform a double-limb heel rise, and is unable to perform a single-limb heel rise. There is a positive "too many toes" sign. There may be significant rearfoot arthritis. Pain is noted medially, and also can be lateral, owing to impingement of lateral talar process.[10] Extra-articular osteotomies may be attempted to treat this stage; however, serious consideration should be given to fusion of the talonavicular and/or subtalar joint (**Fig. 3**).

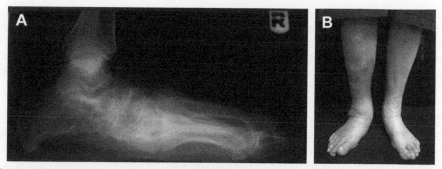

Fig. 3. (*A*) Lateral radiograph showing significant hindfoot and midfoot arthrosis. (*B*) Clinical view of a patient who experiences stage III posterior tibial dysfunction on the right side.

Stage IV deformities are a progression of stage III, with associated tibiotalar valgus and possible arthrosis as a result of the prolonged hindfoot valgus.[11] The treatment of stage IV pes planovalgus is the same as for stage III; however, pain in the ankle joint must also be addressed by means of cautious monitoring, cartilage repair, fusion, or total ankle arthroplasty (**Fig. 4**).

It should be noted that this classification system is mentioned to provide an organized and categorized system to define the stages of the deformity. Clinicians must realize that there can be much overlap of findings from one stage to another, and there exists a spectrum of underlying abnormalities between these stages.

Other classification systems that describe the disorders associated with the dysfunction of the posterior tibial tendon also exist, but are beyond the scope of this article. The reader is encouraged to consult the corresponding references for more detail.[12,13]

OPERATIVE MANAGEMENT

For the purposes of this review, the authors focus here on the operative management of stage II deformities. The adult flexible flatfoot deformity is often the direct result of

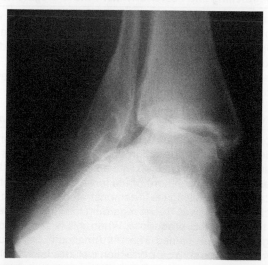

Fig. 4. AP view of ankle showing medial deltoid insufficiency with a posterior tibial tendon dysfunction, stage IV.

dysfunction of the posterior tibial tendon, and eventually the deformity leads to changes in the soft tissues of the medial longitudinal arch. Past surgical approaches included midfoot and hindfoot arthrodesis, and more recent literature suggests the transfer of the flexor digitorum longus tendon combined with a medial calcaneal osteotomy. In addition, some investigators are suggesting the use of a subtalar arthroereisis implant as a potential alternative for the correction of hindfoot valgus.

Isolated Flexor Digitorum Longus Transfer to Navicular

Although this procedure has been described in the past, without correction of the structural abnormalities in the hindfoot, any pure soft-tissue procedure cannot withstand the long-term valgus stress placed on the foot.[12,14–16]

Medial Calcaneal Slide Osteotomy and Posterior Tibial Tendon Augmentation

The osteotomy is commonly done to protect the tendon transfer by improving the supinatory capacity of the gastrocsoleus complex.[17] Brodsky[18] noted significant improvements in the postoperative gait analysis for patients undergoing medial calcaneal osteotomies in conjunction with flexor digitorum longus transfer to the navicular tuberosity. He specifically noted improvements in cadence, stride length, and ankle push-off. Furthermore, studies by Myerson,[19] Fayzi and colleagues,[20] Wacker and colleagues,[21] Guyton and colleagues,[22] and Sammarco and Hockenbury[23] demonstrated a high rate of successful results with short to intermediate follow-up. These studies were mostly level IV case series, but nonetheless demonstrated predictably good outcomes.

These studies do not explain the extent to which the flexor digitorum longus transfer is involved in maintaining longitudinal arch correction, specifically on a long-term basis. There is no way to determine whether the calcaneal slide osteotomy, which offloads the medial column and creates a medializing pull of the Achilles tendon, causes the pain reduction or if the transferred tendon contributes to a reduction in pain.

Lateral Column Lengthening and Posterior Tibial Tendon Augmentation

This procedure was originally described in the pediatric population, using a tricortical graft.[24] Correction of the deformity is accomplished by adducting and plantarflexing the midfoot around the talar head. Hinterman and colleagues[25] and Toolan and colleagues[26] reported promising results in their case series. However, complications of forefoot varus, lateral column overload, nonunion, and graft failure have been reported in other level IV studies.

Double Calcaneal Osteotomies and Posterior Tibial Tendon Augmentation

The combination of the Evans calcaneal osteotomy and the medializing calcaneal slide osteotomy provides a powerful correction and further decreases the load on the posterior-medial structures in comparison with a single osteotomy. In doing so, there is also improvement in overall alignment of the forefoot and midfoot in relation to the hindfoot. Moseir-LaClair and colleagues[27] demonstrated this point in their case series. However, no direct conclusion was drawn regarding the individual benefit of the flexor digitorum longus transfer in this procedure. When this is combined with a posterior group lengthening it has been named The "All American" procedure, as described by Manoli and Pomeroy.[28] The surgical correction includes lateral column lengthening, medializing calcaneal slide osteotomy, flexor digitorum longus transfer to the navicular, and posterior group lengthening.

SURGICAL APPROACH AND EXPERIENCE

In patients who do not demonstrate a significant tear, it has been the experience of the authors to not perform a flexor digitorum longus tendon transfer in those who suffer from stage II posterior tibial tendon dysfunction. The choice of procedures focuses on mechanically realignment of the pathologic foot. The postoperative immobilization with the foot and ankle in a corrective position appears to treat the posterior tibial tendon disorder adequately without the need for an invasive procedure. Postoperatively the foot and ankle are cast and mechanically maintained in the corrected position. This action removes the abnormal stresses placed on the posterior tibial tendon, and provides an environment for the posterior tibial tendon to remodel in a biomechanically corrected position. It has been the authors' experience that the mechanically corrected foot and ankle now protects the rested and "healed" posterior tendon, and prevents future fatigue and disease in the posterior tendon.

Patients are placed in a supine position on the operating table with general anesthesia administered. An ipsilateral pneumatic thigh tourniquet is used to provide hemostasis. A repeat Silfverskiöld test is performed intraoperatively to confirm clinical testing.[29] In the authors' experience, most patients have presented with isolated gastrocnemius equinus when presenting with a symptomatic posterior tibial tendon dysfunction. The posterior muscle group contracture is addressed by either a gastrocnemius recession (endoscopic or open) in the presence of a gastrocnemius equinus, or a tendoachilles lengthening in the presence of a gastrocsoleus equinus. Extraarticular osteotomies of the hindfoot are then executed via a medializing percutaneous calcaneal displacement osteotomy.[30] A Gigli saw is used to execute the osteotomy using a sequence of 4 stab incisions. Following subperiosteal dissection, the Gigli saw is placed in the desired position and the position confirmed fluoroscopically. The Gigli saw should be in position to exit distal to the calcaneal tuberosity (**Fig. 5**).

The osteotomy is executed, taking care not to violate the plantar soft-tissues structure on the plantar cortical exit. The saw is cut at the skin edge and removed. The osteotomy is then placed in the corrected medialized position. Next, 2 parallel guide wires are placed perpendicular to the osteotomy site in preparation for insertion of

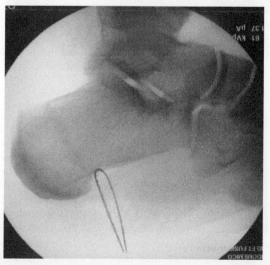

Fig. 5. Intraoperative fluoroscopy showing a percutaneous calcaneal displacement osteotomy.

2 large, partially cancellous screws. Subsequently, the midtarsal joint is evaluated for instability with abduction. If there is no instability, the perpendicular calcaneal osteotomy is fixated with 2 large cancellous screws. If instability is present, an Evans calcaneal osteotomy is performed through an oblique lateral incision, taking care to protect the sural nerve and peroneal tendons. The lengthening is performed with the use of a tricortical allograft. The fixation of choice is large, long, partially threaded cancellous screws. At this point the percutaneous calcaneal osteotomy is fixated first (**Fig. 6**). The first screw inserted is the most superior screw. Insertion is accomplished with typically a short, large, partially threaded cancellous screw, ensuring that the threaded portion of the screw is distal to the osteotomy, resulting in interfragmentary compression of the osteotomy. Next, the authors use a dual-function technique for which the inferior screw is a long, partially threaded cancellous screw.[31] This screw is used to compress the inferior aspect of the percutaneous calcaneal osteotomy and also serves as a positional screw in the distal segment of the Evans calcaneal osteotomy. The purpose of this maneuver is to maintain the length of the Evans osteotomy while providing interfragmentary compression to the percutaneous calcaneal osteotomy site. This technique provides a significant amount of correction, with minimal dissection to the soft tissues and the use of intramedullary fixation. The use of intrafragmentary fixation preserves the soft-tissue structures and prevents the potential complications of painful palpable hardware on the lateral aspect of the calcaneus, and negates the need for soft-tissue stripping if one fixates the Evans osteotomy with a laterally based plate (**Fig. 7**).

If necessary, the medial column is then addressed. In cases where a forefoot varus, osteoarthritis, or instability/hypermobility is identified, the surgeon must recognize which joint or joints of the medial column are involved. The abnormality is corrected by stabilizing the affected joints with an arthrodesis. The goal of the arthrodesis is to adduct and plantarflex the abducted foot into an anatomic position, creating a plantigrade foot, and to reestablish the tripod effect (**Fig. 8**).

The posterior muscle lengthening, a single or double calcaneal osteotomy, and the medial column fusion allow the surgeon to preserve the essential joints. This technique

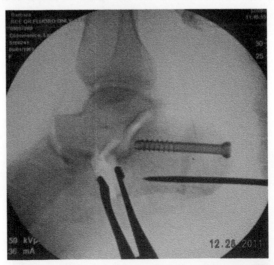

Fig. 6. Lateral intraoperative projection showing fixation of the percutaneous calcaneal osteotomy with interfragmentary compression (superior screw). A guide wire is inserted in preparation for insertion of a dual-function screw across the Evans calcaneal osteotomy.

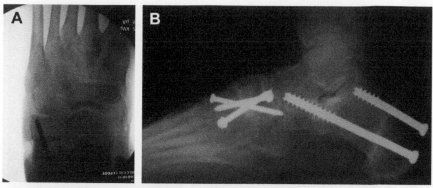

Fig. 7. (*A*) An anterior to posterior guide wire inserted in preparation for a dual-function screw. Note the intramedullary fixation of the Evans calcaneal osteotomy. (*B*) Postoperative lateral radiograph showing the dual-function screw. This screw serves as a positional screw around the Evans osteotomy and an interfragmentary compression screw at the site of the percutaneous calcaneal osteotomy.

provides a stable plantigrade foot and places the foot into anatomic alignment, providing mechanical advantage and eliminating the abnormal stress to the posterior tibial tendon (**Figs. 9** and **10**).

Postoperative care consists of a compressive postoperative bandage and a uni-valve postoperative cast with an anterior evacuation.[32] At 2 weeks the plaster cast is exchanged for a below-the-knee fiberglass cast, which is worn for approximately 4 more weeks as determined by postoperative radiographs. The patient is then

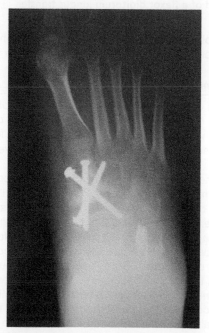

Fig. 8. Postoperative AP radiograph showing a navicular-cuneiform arthrodesis to stabilize the medial column.

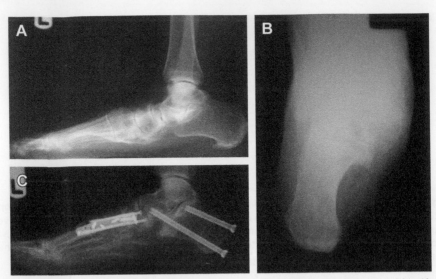

Fig. 9. (*A*) Preoperative lateral projection showing malalignment of midfoot and hindfoot causing abnormal forces along the posterior tibial dysfunction. (*B*) Preoperative view of hindfoot alignment showing a calcaneal valgus, resulting in abnormal forces that lead to a posterior tibial tendon dysfunction. (*C*) Postoperative lateral radiograph showing the foot of a patient who underwent an endoscopic gastrocnemius recession, a percutaneous calcaneal displacement osteotomy, an Evans calcaneal osteotomy, and a midfoot fusion. Note the realignment of the midfoot and hindfoot, therefore decreasing the stress to the posterior tibial tendon. Surgery was not performed on the posterior tibial tendon, and the biomechanically realigned foot provides adequate support to the posterior tibial tendon without the need of a flexor digitorum longus transfer.

transitioned to a controlled ankle motion boot (CAM), and physical therapy is instituted. The patient is then transitioned to regular shoe gear as tolerated.

Lack of Flexor Digitorum Longus Transfer

In the authors' previous case series of 34 patients, considerable radiographic correction was accomplished in performing extra-articular hindfoot osteotomies as well as medial column fusions. Without performing a flexor digitorum longus tendon transfer, patients demonstrated successful postoperative outcomes over an average follow-up period of 14 months.[33]

Many surgeons augment the repair with a flexor digitorum longus tendon transfer to restore and attempt to recreate the function of the posterior tibial tendon. Some surgeons follow a school of thought advising to resect the "diseased" posterior tibial tendon to remove degenerative tissue. Valderrabano and colleagues[34] suggest that this may not always be necessary. These investigators performed MRI analysis of the posterior tibial tendon in patients who underwent flatfoot reconstruction. The study revealed although fatty degeneration of the posterior tibial muscle was present in all patients preoperatively, there was a decrease in degeneration with increasing strength of the posterior tibial muscle and muscular size postoperatively. In addition, they established that the recovery potential of the posterior tibial muscle was significant even after delayed repair of a diseased tendon. Valderrabano and colleagues[34] suggested that the posterior tibial tendon should not be transected because it precludes the recovery potential of the posterior tibial muscle.

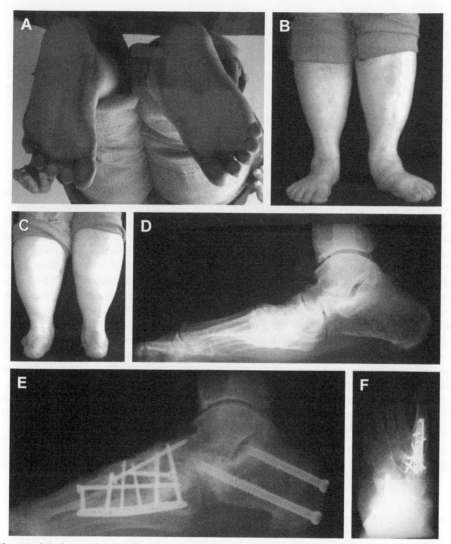

Fig. 10. (*A*) This patient suffers from posterior tibial tendon dysfunction. Note the flatfoot deformity and the forefoot abduction on the hindfoot. (*B*, *C*) Clinical views showing calcaneal valgus and forefoot abduction on a patient who suffers from posterior tibial tendon dysfunction. (*D*) Preoperative lateral projection showing a decrease in the calcaneal pitch, increase in the talar declination, and significant midfoot arthrosis. (*E*, *F*) Postoperative lateral and AP projections following an endoscopic gastrocnemius recession, a percutaneous calcaneal displacement osteotomy, an Evans calcaneal osteotomy, and a midfoot fusion. Note that a flexor digitorum longus tendon transfer was not performed; note also the positive changes in the calcaneal pitch angle, the talar declination, and Kite angle. The essential joints are free and function well, whereas the nonessential joints are fused in the midfoot.

By addressing the structural abnormality at the apex of the deformity, the stress on the posterior tibial tendon was significantly improved. It has been proved in cadaveric studies that realigning the hindfoot can decrease the elongating strain on the posterior tibial tendon by 51%.[35] The load applied on the foot is redirected as the medial longitudinal arch is stabilized, while preserving essential motion at the hindfoot. By positioning the heel in rectus alignment with the leg, the abnormal pull of the tendoachilles and mechanical advantage of the peroneus brevis is eliminated. Another important advantage of avoiding the flexor digitorum longus tendon transfer is the decreased duration of surgery in addition to decreasing the postoperative morbidity of the soft-tissue dissection. During the postoperative period of non–weight bearing and immobilization, the posterior tibial tendon can remodel. This decision is both patient and surgeon friendly for the following reasons:

1. Less operating time
2. Fewer incision sites
3. Reduction of postoperative edema

Ultimately, the use of flexor digitorum longus tendon transfers for posterior tibial tendon augmentation in flatfoot deformity correction has been well documented in the foot and ankle literature; however, the exact role of these transfers in the overall deformity correction still remains an area of debate. There is no proof that structural support can be predictably reproduced with these tendon transfers alone. The authors offer a different perspective, and advocate bony reconstruction of the deformity to establish a biomechanically stable and functional foot and ankle. Rather than performing the tendon transfer, the authors choose to offload the posterior tibial tendon by creating a plantigrade, balanced foot and ankle. As these patients return to full activity and weight bearing, the foot and ankle is mechanically balanced. This balance removes the stress that caused the initial symptoms by neutralizing and realigning the heel under the tibia, placing the midfoot and forefoot in alignment with the hindfoot and relieving the equinus stress of the gastrocnemius and/or soleus. Physical therapy also plays a substantial role in the recovery from this surgery postoperatively.

The authors believe that with an anatomic approach to stage II posterior tibial tendon dysfunction, the need for tendon transfers or major hindfoot fusions is negated, saving operating time for the surgeon and recovery time for the patient.

REFERENCES

1. Key JA. Partial rupture of the tendon of the posterior tibial muscle. J Bone Joint Surg Am 1953;35A(4):1006–8.
2. Hadfield MH, Snyder JW, Liacouras PC, et al. Effects of medializing calcaneal osteotomy on Achilles tendon lengthening and plantar foot pressures. Foot Ankle Int 2003;24(7):523–9.
3. Hiller L, Pinney SJ. Surgical treatment of acquired flatfoot deformity: what is the state of practice among academic foot and ankle surgeons in 2002? Foot Ankle Int 2003;24(9):701–5.
4. Kelikian AS. Sarrafian's anatomy of the foot and ankle. Chapter 5. 3rd edition. Philadelphia: Lippincott Williams and Wilkins; 2011.
5. Brushøj C, Henriksen BM, Albrecht-Beste E, et al. Reproducibility of ultrasound and magnetic resonance imaging measurements of tendon size. Acta Radiol 2006;47(9):954–9.
6. Mickle KJ, Nester CJ, Crofts G, et al. Reliability of ultrasound to measure morphology of the toe flexor muscles. J Foot Ankle Res 2013;6:12.
7. Otis JC, Gage T. Function of the posterior tibial tendon muscle. Foot Ankle Clin 2001;6(1):1–14.
8. Bare AA, Haddad SL. Tenosynovitis of the posterior tibial tendon. Foot Ankle Clin 2001;6(1):37–66.

9. Deland JT, deAsla RJ, Sung IH, et al. Posterior tibial tendon insufficiency: which ligaments are involved? Foot Ankle Int 2005;26(6):427–35.
10. Johnson KA, Strom DE. Tibialis posterior tendon dysfunction. Clin Orthop Relat Res 1989;(239):197–206.
11. Myerson MS, Bluman EM. Stage IV posterior tibial tendon rupture. Foot Ankle Clin 2007;12(2):341–62.
12. Conti S, Michelson J, Jahss M. Clinical significance of magnetic resonance imaging in preoperative planning for reconstruction of posterior tibial tendon ruptures. Foot Ankle Int 1992;13:208–14.
13. Funk DA, Cass JR, Johnson KA. Acquired adult flat foot secondary to posterior tibial-tendon pathology. J Bone Joint Surg Am 1986;68(1):95–102.
14. Jahss MH. Tendon disorders of the foot and ankle. In: Jahss MH, editor. Disorders of the foot and ankle. Medical and surgical management. Philadelphia: W. B. Saunders; 1991. p. 1461–513.
15. Ouzounian TJ. Late flexor digitorum longus tendon rupture after transfer for posterior tibial tendon insufficiency: a case report. Foot Ankle Int 1995;16:519–21.
16. Pomeroy GC, Pike RH, Beals TC, et al. Acquired flatfoot in adults due to dysfunction of the posterior tibial tendon. J Bone Joint Surg Am 1999;81:1173–82.
17. Otis JC, Deland JT, Kenneally S, et al. Medial arch strain after medial displacement calcaneal osteotomy: an in vitro study. Foot Ankle Int 1999;20:222–6.
18. Brodsky JW. Preliminary gait analysis results after posterior tibial tendon reconstruction: a prospective study. Foot Ankle Int 2004;25:96–100.
19. Myerson MS. Adult acquired flatfoot deformity: treatment of dysfunction of the posterior tibial tendon. J Bone Joint Surg Am 1996;78:780–92.
20. Fayzi AH, Nguyen HV, Juliano PJ. Intermediate term follow-up of calcaneal osteotomy and flexor digitorum longus transfer for treatment of posterior tibial tendon dysfunction. Foot Ankle Int 2002;23:1107–11.
21. Wacker JT, Hennessy MS, Saxby TS. Calcaneal osteotomy and transfer of the tendon of the flexor digitorum longus for stage II dysfunction of tibialis posterior: three to five year results. J Bone Joint Surg Br 2002;84(1):54–8.
22. Guyton GP, Jeng C, Krieger LE, et al. Flexor digitorum longus transfer and medial displacement calcaneal osteotomy for posterior tibial tendon dysfunction: a middle term clinical follow-up. Foot Ankle Int 2001;22:627–32.
23. Sammarco GJ, Hockenbury RT. Treatment of stage II posterior tibial tendon dysfunction with flexor hallucis longus transfer and medial displacement calcaneal osteotomy. Foot Ankle Int 2001;22:305–12.
24. Evans D. Calcaneo-valgus deformity. J Bone Joint Surg Br 1975;57:270–8.
25. Hinterman B, Valderrabano V, Kundert HP. Lengthening of the lateral column and reconstruction of the medial soft tissue for treatment of acquired flatfoot deformity associated with insufficiency of the posterior tibial tendon. Foot Ankle Int 1999;20:622–9.
26. Toolan BC, Sangeorzan BJ, Hansen ST. Complex reconstruction for treatment of dorsolateral peritalar subluxation of the foot. Early results after distraction arthrodesis of the calcaneocuboid joint in conjunction with stabilization of and transfer of the flexor digitorum longus tendon, to the midfoot to treat acquired pes planovalgus in adults. J Bone Joint Surg Am 1999;81:1545–60.
27. Moseir-LaClair S, Pomeroy G, Manoli A. Intermediate follow-up on the double osteotomy and tendon transfer procedure for stage II posterior tibial tendon insufficiency. Foot Ankle Int 2001;22:283–91.
28. Pomeroy GC, Manoli A 2nd. A new operative approach for flatfoot secondary to posterior tibial tendon insufficiency: a preliminary report. Foot Ankle Int 1997;18(4):206–12.

29. Silfverskiöld N. Reduction of the uncrossed two-joint muscles of the leg to one-joint muscles in spastic conditions. Acta Chir Scand 1924;56:315.
30. DiDomenico LA, Dull JM. Percutaneous displacement calcaneal osteotomy. J Foot Ankle Surg 2004;43(5):336–7.
31. DiDomenico L, Haro A, Cross D. Double calcaneal osteotomy using single, dual-function screw fixation technique. J Foot Ankle Surg 2011;50:1–3.
32. DiDomenico LA, Sann P. Univalve split plaster cast for postoperative immobilization in foot and ankle surgery. J Foot Ankle Surg 2013;52(2):260–2.
33. DiDomenico LA, Stein DY, Wargo-Dorsey M. Treatment of posterior tibial tendon dysfunction without flexor digitorum tendon transfer: a retrospective study of 34 patients. J Foot Ankle Surg 2011;50:293–8.
34. Valderrabano V, Hintermann B, Wischer T, et al. Recovery of the posterior tibial muscle after late reconstruction following tendon rupture. Foot Ankle Int 2004; 25(2):85–95.
35. Graham ME, Jawrani NT, Goel VK. Effect of extra-osseous talotarsal stabilization on posterior tibial tendon strain in hyperpronating feet. J Foot Ankle Surg 2011; 50:676–81.

Forefoot Supinatus

Erica L. Evans, DPM*, Alan R. Catanzariti, DPM

KEYWORDS

- Forefoot supinatus • Forefoot varus • Pronation • Ankle equinus

KEY POINTS

- The two main mechanisms that contribute to the development of forefoot supinatus are ankle equinus and excessive subtalar joint pronation.
- If the patient fails to respond to nonoperative treatment, or if the patient has a rigid deformity that is not adequately addressed with an orthosis, surgical intervention should be considered.
- For adult acquired flatfoot deformity, there are numerous surgical options that include tendon repair, tendon transfer, osteotomies, arthrodesis, arthroeresis, and combinations of these procedures.
- The operative procedures chosen to address the etiology of the adult acquired flatfoot must address all the components of the deformity to restore proper balance and function.
- Failure to recognize and correct any residual forefoot supinatus deformity following hindfoot realignment may lead to failure and recurrence of the flatfoot deformity.

The adult acquired flatfoot deformity (AAFD) is one of the most common disorders seen by foot and ankle specialists. A flatfoot is characterized by abduction and supination of the forefoot with a collapsed medial longitudinal arch. However, the relationships between the osseous and soft tissue structures that contribute to a deformity often vary in degree of severity, nature, and location of pain and instability.[1]

The supination of the forefoot that develops with adult acquired flatfoot is defined as forefoot supinatus. This deformity is an acquired soft tissue adaptation in which the forefoot is inverted on the rearfoot. The degree of forefoot supinatus present in an individual patient is the function of calcaneal eversion, the chronicity of the problem, and adaptive muscle and osseous changes. When significant adaptive alteration in muscle, ligament, and articular surfaces has developed over an extended period of time, the supinatus may become fixed and difficult to differentiate from forefoot varus.[2]

Forefoot supinatus can mimic, and often be mistaken for, a forefoot varus, which likely contributes to these two terms incorrectly being used interchangeably. A forefoot varus differs from forefoot supinatus in that a forefoot varus is a congenital

Foot & Ankle Institute, Foot & Ankle Surgery, West Penn Hospital, 4800 Friendship Avenue, N1, Pittsburgh, PA 15224, USA
* Corresponding author.
E-mail address: eevans1@wpahs.org

Clin Podiatr Med Surg 31 (2014) 405–413
http://dx.doi.org/10.1016/j.cpm.2014.03.009
0891-8422/14/$ – see front matter © 2014 Elsevier Inc. All rights reserved.

osseous deformity that induces subtalar joint pronation, whereas forefoot supinatus is acquired and develops because of subtalar joint pronation. This article concentrates on the acquired form of forefoot supinatus.

ETIOLOGY

Supination of the foot around the longitudinal axis of the midtarsal joint is required to accommodate normal calcaneal eversion in gait (4–6 degrees). When excessive calcaneal eversion is present, excessive inversion of the foot about the longitudinal midtarsal joint axis is the usual corollary finding. In addition to longitudinal axis supinatory subluxation, dorsal displacement of the first ray also occurs with calcaneal eversion as the result of first ray hypermobility.[2]

Forefoot supinatus is a compensatory deformity that develops secondarily to pathologic forces that tend to cause dorsiflexion or prevent plantarflexion of the metatarsals. There are two main mechanisms recognized that contribute to the development of a forefoot supinatus deformity: ankle equinus and excessive subtalar joint pronation.[3]

Equinus refers to any condition, either structural or functional, that restricts ankle joint dorsiflexion to less than 10 degrees when the subtalar joint is in neutral and the midtarsal joint is fully pronated.[4] Compensation for an ankle equinus typically results in subtalar and midtarsal joint pronation. The Achilles tendon forces the calcaneus into valgus and limits subtalar joint inversion in the presence of equinus.[1] Ankle equinus ultimately results in a direct dorsiflexory force on the metatarsals after the limit of ankle joint dorsiflexion is reached.[3]

The second mechanism responsible for the development of forefoot supinatus is excessive subtalar joint pronation during forefoot loading. The pronated position of the subtalar joint allows for increased pronation of the midtarsal joint. Any additional eversion of the forefoot about the oblique axis of the midtarsal joint must be compensated by further forefoot inversion by dorsiflexion of the medial column.[3]

An unlocked midtarsal joint during midstance allows the concentric contraction of the Achilles tendon to plantarflex the hindfoot on the forefoot. This places significant overload on the posterior tibial tendon and spring ligament, in addition to the long and short plantar ligaments and plantar aponeurosis.[5] This process results in the radiographic finding of "lateral peritalar subluxation."[6] This peritalar subluxation results in midfoot abduction and forefoot supinatus.[1]

Whatever the contribution of each deformity, the result in long-standing cases of calcaneal eversion is a fixed or semi-rigid position of inversion of the forefoot relative to the rearfoot.[2] Both the underlying etiologic factor and the acquired deformity should be addressed when treating a supinatus deformity.

CLINICAL EVALUATION

Before any specific examination for forefoot supinatus, the range of motion of the subtalar, midtarsal, first ray, and first metatarsal phalangeal joints should be evaluated.[2]

The position of the foot required for measuring the forefoot to rearfoot relationship must be maintained for all subsequent measurements. Deformity through the medial column is best evaluated with the patient in the seated position. The hindfoot is placed in a "neutral position" by centering the navicular over the talar head. The deformity is confirmed by palpating the medial border of the foot and the relationship of the navicular tuberosity to the talar head. As the hindfoot is held in this position with one hand, the opposite hand is used to passively bring the ankle to neutral dorsiflexion by placing force on the plantar aspect of the fourth and fifth metatarsal heads. At this point, the relationship of the first and fifth metatarsals are evaluated by viewing the foot "head-on" to determine the degree of elevation of the first ray relative to the fifth ray (**Fig. 1**).[7]

Stability of the first ray is then assessed, again in a seated position, by stabilizing the lesser four metatarsals with one hand and then using the opposite hand to manipulate the first metatarsal. The dorsiflexion and plantarflexion of the first ray in relation to the rest of the foot is assessed while the windlass mechanism is engaged to determine if there is excessive sagittal plane motion or if there is pain or crepitus with range of motion (**Fig. 2**).[8]

RADIOGRAPHIC EVALUATION

In addition to the physical examination, weight-bearing radiographs play an important role in determining and assessing the deformity of the patient's foot. Weight-bearing radiographs of the foot and ankle should be obtained to help provide a comprehensive assessment of forefoot supinatus.

Subluxation of the talonavicular (TN) and naviculocuneiform (NC) joints on anteroposterior views, together with significant superimposition of the lesser tarsus on lateral views, characterizes forefoot supinatus. The major rotational component of the deformity seems to occur at the TN articulation. Because longitudinal axis supination is usually accompanied by simultaneous oblique axis pronation, midtarsal abduction and cuboid abduction are marked on the dorsoplantar radiographs.[2]

On a normal weight-bearing anteroposterior and lateral radiograph, the calcaneocuboid joint should be at the same level as the TN joint. With adult acquired flatfoot, the foot radiographs show the appearance of a short lateral column compared with a medial column, with the TN joint approximately 3 to 5 mm distal to the calcaneocuboid joint.[9]

Further radiographic examination should include careful evaluation of the talar head uncovering, talo–first metatarsal angle, and calcaneal pitch (**Fig. 3**).

In addition to angular measurements, the joints of the medial column should be evaluated on the weight-bearing lateral radiograph. Medial column joints may show evidence of degenerative changes, such as joint space narrowing, subchondral sclerosis, or osteophytes. Identifying an unstable or arthritic medial column joint influences the surgical treatment plan.[8]

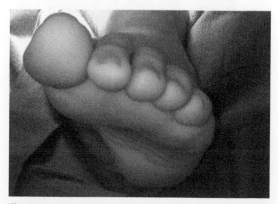

Fig. 1. This picture illustrates the degree of forefoot elevation of the first ray relative to the fifth ray.

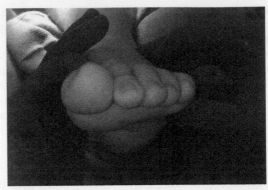

Fig. 2. The forefoot supinatus is reduced by stabilizing the lateral metatarsals and plantar-flexing the first metatarsal with the opposite hand.

FIXED VERSUS REDUCIBLE

The forefoot compensates for many structural abnormalities by dorsiflexion of the medial column. Early in the flatfoot deformity, the medial column remains dorsiflexed only during this compensation; however, as the deformity progresses, soft tissue adaptation results in the medial column remaining dorsiflexed during nonweightbearing.[3]

When articular and muscular adaptive alterations are not permanent in nature, forefoot supinatus should reduce when calcaneal eversion is limited to normal excursion.[10]

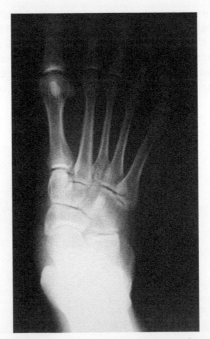

Fig. 3. Preoperative weight-bearing anteroposterior radiograph used to evaluate Talar head uncovering, talo–first metatarsal angle, and calcaneocuboid joint.

Stabilization of the subtalar joint should result in a more effective pronatory influence of the peroneus longus on the longitudinal axis of the midtarsal joint and a greater plantarflexory component on the first ray. When significant adaptive alterations in the articular facets and soft tissues (in particular the tibialis anterior) have occurred, forefoot supinatus fails to reduce, even when etiologic factors have been corrected and excessive calcaneal eversion eliminated. The result is a patient with medial imbalance and a fixed forefoot supinatus deformity.[2] If a forefoot supinatus deformity is not recognized, and a medial column procedure is not performed to help balance an unstable foot, the patient may experience lateral foot pain caused by lateral column overload.[11]

In certain patients that have a flexible or reducible deformity, nonoperative treatment of medial column deformity or instability with a foot orthosis may be helpful. A custom molded semi-rigid foot orthosis or arch support is posted at the medial heel and lateral forefoot to help correct foot pronation and forefoot supinatus.[8]

If the patient fails to respond to nonoperative treatment, or if the patient has a rigid deformity that is not adequately addressed with an orthosis, surgical intervention should be considered.

SURGICAL OPTIONS

When considering surgical procedures for the treatment of forefoot supinatus, it is important to recall that the supinatus deformity is an acquired deformity secondary to an underlying cause of the adult acquired flatfoot.

For AAFD, there are numerous surgical options that include tendon repair, tendon transfer, osteotomies, arthrodesis, arthroeresis, and combinations of these procedures. The operative procedures chosen must address the cause of the adult acquired flatfoot, and most important, must address all the components of the deformity to restore balance and function.[8]

Dorsiflexion and inversion are the main components of forefoot supinatus along the medial column. Various surgical options have been described to address forefoot supinatus through the medial column. The appropriate choice is based on the location of deformity and identification of abnormal or arthritic joints.[8]

Following the clinical and radiographic evaluation, one must determine if the supinatus deformity is reducible or fixed. In addition, when considering the surgical procedures, it is important to take into account the patient's comorbidities, lifestyle demands, and the patient's postoperative expectations.

When the deformity is flexible and not associated with degenerative joint disease, joint-sparing reconstructive osteotomies may be considered. The reconstructive procedures may include medial soft tissue reconstruction that involves the flexor digitorum longus transfer, repair of the posterior tibial tendon, or possible imbrications of the spring ligament if needed.[8]

Osseous procedures indicated for the flexible forefoot supinatus include medial stabilization procedures, such as a Cotton osteotomy (plantarflexion opening wedge medial cuneiform osteotomy). This procedure should be used as an adjunct procedure to reconstruction of a flatfoot deformity. The Cotton osteotomy is primarily used to correct forefoot supinatus with elevation of the medial column where the deformity is located at the first tarsometatarsal (TMT) joint or NC joint. The Cotton osteotomy is a joint-sparing procedure; thus, the first TMT joint should be stable or have only mild instability on physical examination. There should not be any radiographic evidence of joint abnormality, such as plantar gapping on the lateral weight-bearing radiograph or findings of significant osteoarthritis. The authors perform the Cotton osteotomy as a last step in surgical reconstruction of the AAFD. Hindfoot realignment unmasks the magnitude of supinatus. This is important when determining the amount of correction that is required to address the deformity. The Cotton osteotomy has proved to be useful in correcting residual forefoot supinatus in AAFD and should be carefully considered when there is no abnormality at the first TMT joint (**Fig. 4**).[8]

Lutz and Myerson[12] state that a medial column opening wedge osteotomy, when used as part of the surgical management of a symptomatic flatfoot with forefoot supinatus, has been shown to radiographically correct the forefoot supinatus and provide medial column stability. A medial column procedure is helpful in stabilizing the joints and bridging the forefoot into a plantigrade position.[13] Failure to recognize and correct any residual forefoot supinatus deformity following hindfoot realignment may lead to failure and recurrence of the flatfoot deformity.[12] If the forefoot remains supinated and a medial column procedure is not performed, the hindfoot must evert to maintain forefoot alignment. Therefore, this hindfoot eversion may lead to failure of the flatfoot corrective procedures.[12]

When the supinatus deformity is rigid or associated with moderate to severe degenerative joint disease, the authors consider arthrodesis procedures to appropriately address the deformity. Medial column arthrodesis' are versatile procedures for the correction of AAFDs when forefoot supinatus or medial column instability is present.[14] These procedures include arthrodesis of the first TMT joint, or more proximal procedures including NC or TN arthrodesis.

First TMT arthrodesis is indicated to address medial column instability secondary to AAFD. Much like other medial column procedures, first TMT arthrodesis should be used as an adjunct to a comprehensive flatfoot reconstruction. It is indicated to address residual forefoot supinatus and medial column instability in the AAFD, especially when the deformity includes the first TMT joint. If significant forefoot supinatus remains following appropriate hindfoot correction, with associated instability, hypermobility, or degenerative changes at the first TMT joint, a first TMT arthrodesis should be considered to address forefoot supinatus.[8]

Medial column instability may also exist at the level of the NC or TN joint.[8] The NC joint arthrodesis may provide significant correction in the transverse and sagittal planes. Arthrodesis enhances the windlass mechanism's ability to plantarflex and adduct the forefoot on the hindfoot, correcting the residual forefoot supinatus deformity.[15] Because the NC joint is often implicated in medial column instability, arthrodesis is considered an effective means of addressing the fault and hypermobility without compromising normal foot function.[16] NC arthrodesis is used in conjunction with other osseous and soft tissue procedures to correct the collapsed flatfoot when there is significant instability present within the medial column.[16] Because the

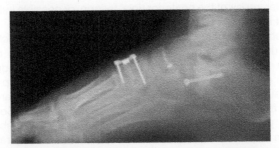

Fig. 4. Postoperative radiograph demonstrating the use of a Cotton osteotomy to correct any residual forefoot supinatus following hindfoot realignment.

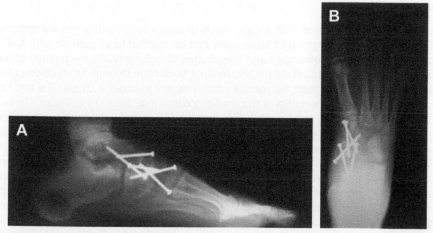

Fig. 5. (*A, B*) Lateral and anteroposterior radiographs with the use of a TN arthrodesis and NC arthrodesis to stabilize the medial column.

NC joint is the center of the lever arm of the foot and is therefore subject to bending-moment stress, concomitant posterior muscle lengthening is recommended (**Fig. 5**).[16]

Medial column deformity and instability may also present more proximal at the TN joint. When instability at the TN joint is secondary to dysfunction of the posterior tibial tendon or collapse of the TN joint, an isolated TN arthrodesis can be considered.[17] This procedure is mostly indicated for a supinatus deformity that is either grossly unstable, or has progressed to a more rigid flatfoot deformity. Although an arthrodesis of the TN joint involves only a single joint, biomechanically it results in almost complete loss of motion in the subtalar and transverse tarsal joints. This motion is lost because for the subtalar joint to invert and evert, the navicular must rotate over the talar head. Thus, if TN movement is restricted, subtalar motion does not occur (**Fig. 6**).[17–19]

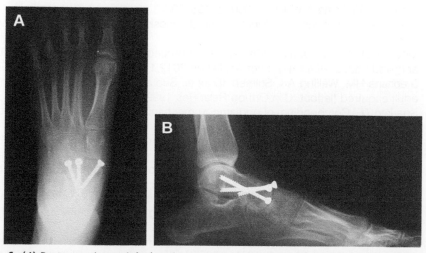

Fig. 6. (*A*) Postoperative weight-bearing anteroposterior and (*B*) lateral radiographs of an isolated TN arthrodesis.

SUMMARY

AAFD is a complex problem with a wide variety of presentation and treatment options. No single procedure or group of procedures can be applied to all patients with AAFD because of the various etiologies and magnitudes of deformity. As the posture of the foot progresses into hindfoot valgus and forefoot abduction through attenuation of the medial structures of the foot, the medial column begins to change shape. The first ray begins to elevate and the joints of the medial column may begin to collapse. Careful physical examination and review of weight-bearing radiographs determines which patients have an associated forefoot supinatus deformity that may require correction at the time of flatfoot reconstruction.[8]

Correction of AAFD may require a combination of soft tissue procedures to restore dynamic inversion power, and osseous procedures to correct the hindfoot and midfoot malalignments. Medial column instability is an important component of flatfoot deformity. Failure to address the medial column instability can result in a biomechanically unstable foot, resulting in residual forefoot deformity.[1] Depending on the deformity, joint-sparing and arthrodesis procedures can address forefoot supinatus as part of a comprehensive approach for correction of the AAFD.

REFERENCES

1. Lee MS, Maker JM. Revision of failed flatfoot surgery. Clin Podiatr Med Surg 2009; 26:47–58.
2. Jacobs AM, Oloff LM. Surgical management of forefoot supinatus in flexible flatfoot deformity. J Foot Surg 1984;23:410–9.
3. Roy KJ, Scherer P. Forefoot supinatus. J Am Podiatr Med Assoc 1986;76:390–4.
4. Bird SR, Black N, Newton P. Sports injuries: causes, diagnosis, treatment and prevention. (United Kingdom): Stanley Thomes Ltd; 1997. p. 50.
5. Richie DH. Biomechanics and clinical analysis of the adult acquired flatfoot. Clin Podiatr Med Surg 2007;24:617–44.
6. Hansen ST. Progressive symptomatic flat foot (lateral peritalar subluxation). In: Hansen ST, editor. Functional reconstruction of the foot and ankle. Philadelphia: Lippincott Williams & Wilkins; 2000. p. 195–207.
7. Alexander IJ. The foot: examination and diagnosis. New York: Churchill Livingston; 1990.
8. McCormick JJ, Johnson JE. Medial column procedures in the correction of adult acquired flatfoot deformity. Foot Ankle Clin 2012;17:283–98.
9. Stephens HM, Walling AK, Solmen JD, et al. Subtalar repositional arthrodesis of adult acquired flatfoot. Clin Orthop Relat Res 1999;(365):69–73.
10. Sgarlato TE. Compendium of podiatric biomechanics. California College of Podiatric Medicine; 1973.
11. Deland JT. Adult acquired flatfoot deformity. J Am Acad Orthop Surg 2008;16: 399–406.
12. Lutz M, Myerson M. Radiographic analysis of an opening wedge osteotomy of the medial cuneiform. Foot Ankle Int 2011;32:278–87.
13. Benthien RA, Parks BG, Guyton GP, et al. Lateral column calcaneal lengthening, flexor digitorum longus transfer, and opening wedge medial cuneiform osteotomy for flexible flatfoot: a biomechanical study. Foot Ankle Int 2007;28:70–7.
14. Catanzariti AR, Mendicino RW, Maskill MP. McGlamry's comprehensive textbook of foot and ankle surgery. Posterior tibial tendon dysfunction. Philadelphia: Lippincott Williams & Wilkins; 2013. p. 636–69.

15. Bundy AM, Grossman JP. Naviculocuneiform arthrodesis. Clin Podiatr Med Surg 2007;24:753–63.
16. Ford LA, Hamilton GA. Naviculocuneiform arthrodesis. Clin Podiatr Med Surg 2004;21:141–56.
17. Coughlin MN, Mann RA, Saltzman CL. Surgery of the foot and ankle. Arthrodesis of the foot and ankle. Philadelphia: Mosby Elsevier; 2007. p. 1087–123.
18. Elftman H. The transverse tarsal joint and its control. Clin Orthop 1960;16:41.
19. O'Malley MJ, Deland JT, Lee K. Selective hindfoot arthrodesis for the treatment of adult acquired flatfoot deformity: an in vitro study. Foot Ankle Int 1995;16:411–7.

Triple Arthrodesis for Adult Acquired Flatfoot

Alan R. Catanzariti, DPM[a],*, Brian T. Dix, DPM[a], Phillip E. Richardson, DPM[a], Robert W. Mendicino, DPM[b,c]

KEYWORDS

- Adult acquired flatfoot • Triple arthrodesis • Image intensification • Bone graft

KEY POINTS

- The primary goal of triple arthrodesis for stage III and IV adult acquired flatfoot is to obtain a well-aligned plantigrade foot that will support the ankle in optimal alignment.
- Ancillary procedures including posterior muscle group lengthening, medial displacement calcaneal osteotomy, medial column stabilization, peroneus brevis tenotomy, or transfer and harvest of regional bone graft are often necessary to achieve adequate realignment.
- Image intensification is helpful in confirming optimal realignment before fixation.
- Results of triple arthrodesis are enhanced with adequate preparation of joint surfaces, bone graft/orthobiologics, 2-point fixation of all 3 tritarsal joints, and a vertical heel position.

Triple arthrodesis for adult acquired flatfoot is typically indicated in stage III and stage IV deformities.[1–4] These patients often have end-stage arthritis and significant deformity that is nonreducible. The authors also consider triple arthrodesis when there has been a failed joint-sparing procedure or a failed arthrodesis of an isolated tritarsal joint to address stage II adult acquired flatfoot. The goals of surgery include resolution of symptoms, realignment, and sound arthrodesis.

Acceptable outcomes following triple arthrodesis in stage III adult acquired flatfoot are based on the surgeon's ability to obtain a plantigrade foot that will support the ankle in optimal alignment. Therefore, realignment becomes the most important factor relative to good results. A well-aligned triple arthrodesis will result in normal physiologic contact pressures throughout the ankle, and prevent medial soft-tissue attenuation and ensuing degenerative changes. A triple arthrodesis with residual valgus deformity predisposes the ankle to attenuation of medial soft-tissue constraints and subsequent valgus deformity in addition to degenerative joint disease.

[a] Division of Foot & Ankle Surgery, West Penn Hospital, 4800 Friendship Avenue, Pittsburgh, PA 15224, USA; [b] OhioHealth Orthopedic Surgeons, Hilliard, OH, USA; [c] Foot & Ankle Surgical Residency, West Penn Hospital, 4800 Friendship Avenue, Pittsburgh, PA 15224, USA
* Corresponding author.
E-mail address: acatanzariti@faiwp.com

Clin Podiatr Med Surg 31 (2014) 415–433
http://dx.doi.org/10.1016/j.cpm.2014.03.004
0891-8422/14/$ – see front matter © 2014 Elsevier Inc. All rights reserved.

Preoperative imaging should include weight-bearing radiographs of the foot and ankle, hindfoot alignment/long-leg calcaneal axial radiographs, and advanced imaging. Weight-bearing radiographs of the ankle are necessary to evaluate the presence of valgus deformity and degenerative changes. Long-leg calcaneal axial and hindfoot alignment views provide information regarding frontal alignment. The authors sometimes consider magnetic resonance imaging (MRI) to evaluate the ankle arthritis that might be equivocal on standard radiographs. In addition, when the foot deformity is somewhat severe and the ankle is congruent on an anteroposterior (AP) radiograph, an MRI is obtained to evaluate the deltoid ligament. In such situations whereby the deltoid ligament is attenuated on MRI, the authors will consider as adjunct procedures a medial displacement osteotomy to offload the deltoid ligament, and deltoid repair.

Several ancillary procedures are necessary to obtain a plantigrade foot. Posterior muscle group lengthening, in the form of either an Achilles tendon lengthening or gastrocnemius recession, is invariably required in stage III adult acquired flatfoot. The authors use gastrocnemius recession in most cases. However, following realignment of a severe deformity, an Achilles tendon lengthening may be necessary to obtain adequate length and restore sagittal plane position.

Medial displacement osteotomy of the calcaneus has been mentioned previously as an adjunct procedure to address ankle valgus or medial soft-tissue attenuation (**Fig. 1**). Resnick and colleagues[5] have shown that a triple arthrodesis in

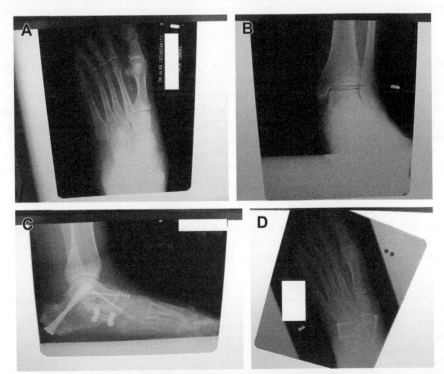

Fig. 1. (*A*) Anteroposterior (AP) radiograph of flatfoot deformity. (*B*) AP radiograph of the ankle, showing valgus deformity. (*C, D*) Postoperative radiographs of triple arthrodesis combined with medial displacement osteotomy to address valgus deformity of the ankle.

combination with a medial displacement osteotomy of the calcaneus will reduce deltoid ligament forces by 56%. Song and colleagues[6] have also suggested that medializing the calcaneus following triple arthrodesis protects the deltoid complex.

The authors will consider medial column stabilization, in the form of either naviculo-cuneiform arthrodesis or first tarsometatarsal arthrodesis, when medial column insta-bility is identified following triple arthrodesis for stage III adult acquired flatfoot (**Fig. 2**). Insufficiency of the medial column can result in a functional varus. Failure to address medial column instability can result in a lateral column overload when patients begin weight bearing, with subsequent fifth metatarsal base bursitis or fifth metatarsal head callosities.

Harvesting of regional bone graft and/or bone marrow aspirate is a part of virtually every triple arthrodesis. Cancellous bone is often harvested from the calcaneus using 6- to 8-mm trephines through small lateral incisions (**Fig. 3**). Bone marrow aspirate is obtained from the calcaneus before tourniquet inflation. The cancellous bone is packed into arthrodesis sites. The extra-articular areas along the undersurface of the talus and the dorsal surface of the calcaneus are decorticated. The bone marrow aspirate is mixed with bioactive glass and is then packed into this extra-articular area.

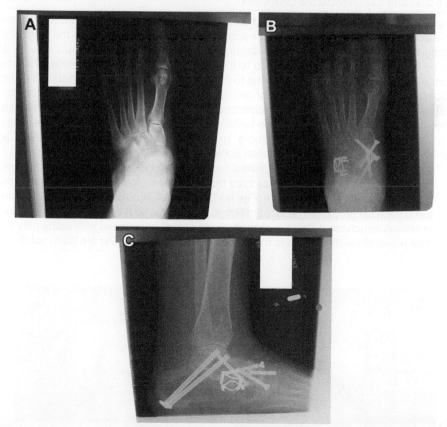

Fig. 2. (*A*) Preoperative AP radiograph. (*B*, *C*) Postoperative radiographs of triple arthrodesis with naviculocuneiform arthrodesis to address medial column instability.

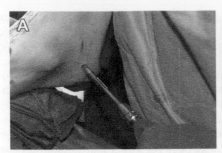
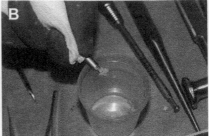

Fig. 3. (*A, B*) Harvesting of small, cancellous bone grafts.

Transfer of peroneus brevis to peroneus longus tendon is performed when the deformity is severe (**Fig. 4**). Severe contracture of the peroneus brevis tendon can sometimes make it difficult to obtain complete realignment. As an alternative, the authors sometimes transect both tendons.

SURGICAL TECHNIQUE FOR TRIPLE ARTHRODESIS
Subtalar and Calcaneocuboid Dissection

Triple arthrodesis is usually performed under general anesthesia; however, these procedures may also be performed with spinal anesthesia depending on the patient's comorbidities and overall medical status. The patient is positioned supine with a bump placed under the ipsilateral hip to internally rotate the foot and ankle. The patient's heel should be located just distal to the end of the operating room table to allow access to the posterior calcaneus for delivery of fixation and to permit easier manipulation of the extremity during intraoperative imaging. The extremity is elevated on several stacks of towels or a bump to facilitate use of retractors and to enhance imaging during the procedure. The authors typically use a thigh tourniquet, which is released after osteosynthesis has been achieved.

Triple arthrodesis is typically performed through a combination of medial and lateral incisions. The lateral incision extends from the tip of the lateral malleolus and courses distally to the fourth metatarsal base (**Fig. 5**). This incision is dorsal to the peroneal tendons and sural nerve. Care is taken to maintain hemostasis with cauterization or ligation of the venous structures within this area. A sponge lightly moistened with saline may be used for planal dissection down to the fascia. The peroneal tendons are then mobilized

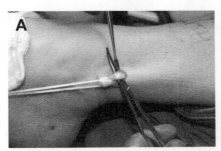
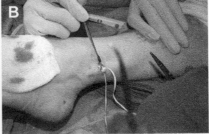

Fig. 4. (*A, B*) Transfer of the peroneus brevis to longus tendon to eliminate abductory pull and contracture of the peroneus brevis tendon.

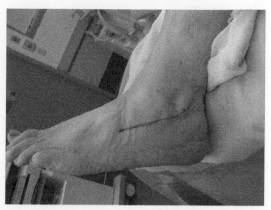

Fig. 5. Lateral incision for triple arthrodesis. Incision begins just proximal to the tip of the malleolus and extends distally to the fourth metatarsal base.

with Metzenbaum scissors and retracted inferiorly (**Fig. 6**). Dissection is then carried down to the level of deep fascia and the extensor digitorum brevis muscle belly. An inverted T-shaped incision is performed with the base of the incision along the inferior aspect of the muscle belly, extending proximally along the lateral capsule of the talocalcaneal joint. The vertical arm of the incision is within the sinus tarsi. A second vertical

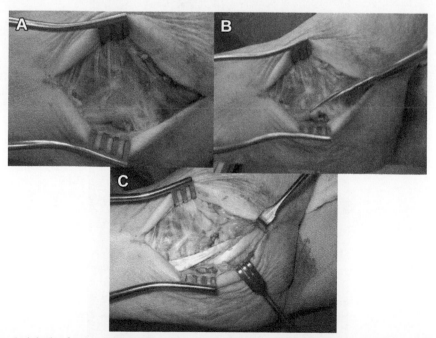

Fig. 6. (*A*) The fascia covering the extensor digitorum muscle belly. The peroneal tendons are inferior and the sinus tarsi is proximal. (*B*) Peroneal tendon sheath being incised with Metzenbaum scissors. (*C*) Exposure of the peroneal tendons for inferior retraction.

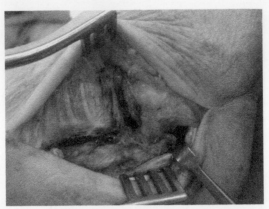

Fig. 7. Inverted-T incision with the vertical within the sinus tarsi, and the horizontal arm along the inferior aspect of the extensor digitorum longus muscle belly and the lateral talocalcaneal joint. Note the soft-tissue resection within the sinus tarsi.

incision is then placed parallel within the sinus tarsi, and the contents of the sinus tarsi are thoroughly evacuated (**Fig. 7**). This action enhances visualization and access to the subtalar joint (STJ). Dissection is then carried proximally along the lateral talocalcaneal joint, where the calcaneofibular ligament is incised to facilitate access to the STJ (**Fig. 8**).

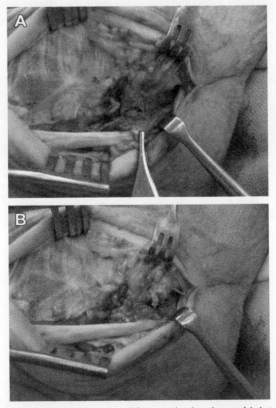

Fig. 8. (*A*) Intact calcaneofibular ligament. (*B*) Lateral talocalcaneal joint following transaction of the calcaneofibular ligament.

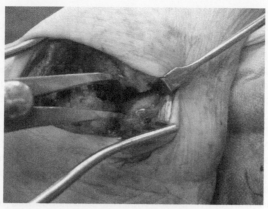

Fig. 9. Lamina spreader within the sinus tarsi exposing the posterior facet of the subtalar joint.

The lateral talocalcaneal ligaments and calcaneofibular ligament are often contracted in long-standing adult acquired flatfoot. Releasing these periarticular structures will enhance mobilization of the STJ, and therefore permit easier access and realignment.

Preparation of Subtalar Joint and Calcaneocuboid Joint

A lamina spreader with teeth is placed within the sinus tarsi, which provides access to the STJ (**Fig. 9**). Alternatively, pin-distractors can be used. The cartilage of the posterior and middle facet is thoroughly removed with the use of narrow, straight, and

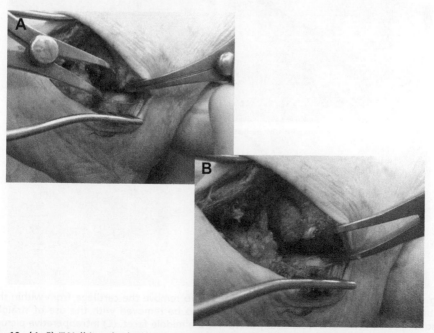

Fig. 10. (*A, B*) "Walking the lamina spreaders" through various areas of the subtalar joint to expose articular surface for cartilage debridement and joint preparation.

curved osteotomes. This process is often tedious but essential. Straight and angled curettes are also beneficial when debriding cartilage from the middle facet of the STJ. Cartilage debris should then be completely removed from within the joint. The authors often "walk the lamina spreaders" throughout the various areas of the STJ to gain access to the entire joint (**Figs. 10** and **11**). The articular cartilage debris is then thoroughly removed from the STJ region before preparing the subchondral plate. The lateral aspect of the talonavicular joint (TNJ) may be visualized from the lateral incision and partially prepared before accessing this joint from the medial incision. The subchondral plates of both the talus and calcaneus are first fenestrated with a 2.5-mm drill and then methodically broken using a straight, narrow osteotome. A small distractor can initially be used to access the STJ when the lamina spreader is too large (**Fig. 12**). The goal of joint preparation is to develop a healthy cancellous substrate that will go on to primary union.

A lamina spreader with teeth is placed within the calcaneocuboid joint, and the same technique as described for cartilage removal and joint preparation is used (**Fig. 13**).

Dissection and Preparation of Talonavicular Joint

The second incision of triple arthrodesis is located medially. This incision begins within the medial gutter of the ankle joint and extends distally to the base of the first metatarsal (**Fig. 14**). The incision provides access to the TNJ and can be extended distally to incorporate the naviculocuneiform and/or first tarsometatarsal joint if necessary.

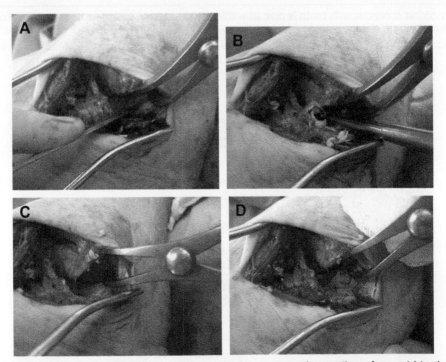

Fig. 11. (*A*) Small straight osteotome being used to remove the cartilage from within the subtalar joint. (*B*) Subtalar joint cartilage can also be removed with the use of straight and angled curettes; this is especially useful for the middle facet. (*C*) Intraoperative picture of the subtalar joint following cartilage removal. (*D*) Methodical breaking of the subchondral plate to enhance arthrodesis.

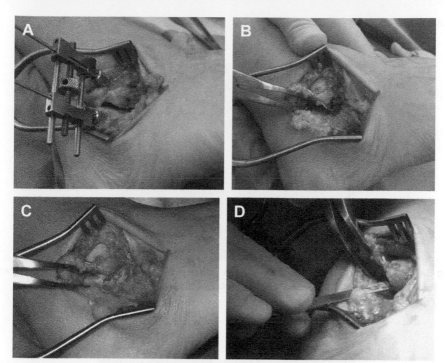

Fig. 12. (*A*) Initial use of a minidistractor to expose the subtalar joint when the lamina spreader is too large. (*B*) Lamina spreader has now been inserted. (*C, D*) Subchondral plate preparation with the use of small osteotomes.

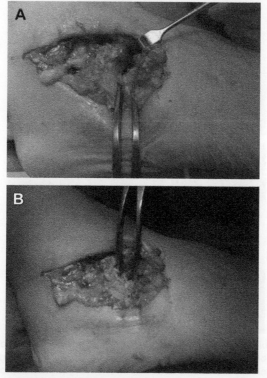

Fig. 13. (*A*) Calcaneocuboid joint following cartilage removal. (*B*) Calcaneocuboid joint following methodical breaking of the subchondral plate.

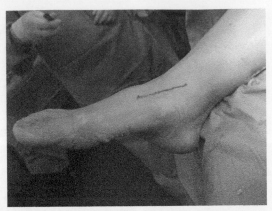

Fig. 14. Medial incision for a triple arthrodesis. This incision begins within the medial gutter of the ankle and extends toward the first metatarsal base.

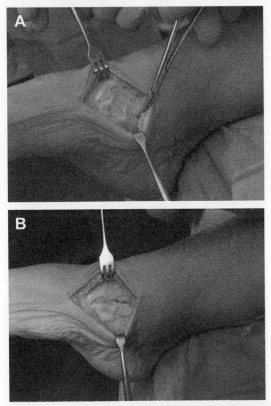

Fig. 15. (*A*) The tibialis anterior tendon is located along the dorsal aspect, and tibialis posterior tendon along the inferior aspect of the wound. (*B*) The deep fascia/periosteal incision is made between the 2 tendons, with care taken to ligate vessels along the most distal aspect of the ankle joint capsule.

There is often a large number of vessels in this area. This stage requires ligation, especially within the distal portion of the ankle capsule. A sponge can be used for planal dissection down to the level of deep fascia. The tibialis anterior tendon is located within the dorsal aspect of the wound and the tibialis posterior tendon within the inferior aspect of the wound. The deep fascia and periosteum should then be incised between these 2 tendons, and all dissection performed in a subperiosteal manner (**Fig. 15**). Dissection must be extended both inferiorly and dorsally to obtain adequate exposure. A lamina spreader or small pin distractor is then used to open the TNJ. The cartilage is removed using a combination of narrow, straight, and curved osteotomes. All cartilage debris should be thoroughly removed from the TNJ (**Fig. 16**). A 2.5-mm drill and a narrow osteotome are then used to break the subchondral plates in a methodical fashion (**Fig. 17**).

Realignment/Positioning and Fixation

The STJ is the first joint to be realigned. The realignment is based on clinical and radiographic assessment. The calcaneus is placed vertical to the lower leg with the STJ in a neutral position. This position is confirmed with an intraoperative axial image, which should show the calcaneus parallel to the tibia (**Fig. 18**). Lateral radiographs should demonstrate restoration of the calcaneal inclination angle (**Fig. 19**). Fixation is accomplished with percutaneous large-diameter cannulated screws. The authors prefer 2-point fixation. The first guide pin is placed from the inferior aspect of the calcaneus

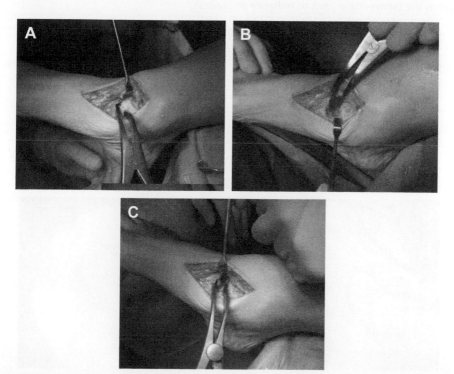

Fig. 16. (*A*) Exposure of the talonavicular joint. (*B*) Talonavicular joint following cartilage removal. (*C*) Talonavicular joint following methodical breaking of the subchondral plate to enhance arthrodesis.

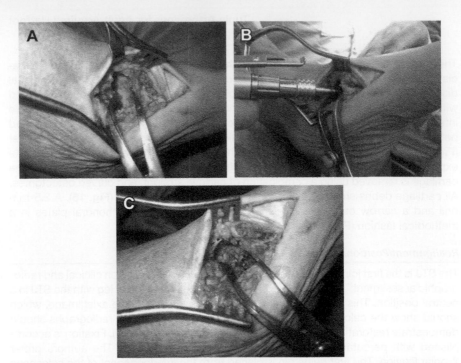

Fig. 17. (*A*) The talonavicular joint following cartilage removal. (*B*) A surgairtome with rotary sidecutter burr being used to prepare the talonavicular joint. (*C*) The bone paste is left within the talonavicular joint to enhance arthrodesis.

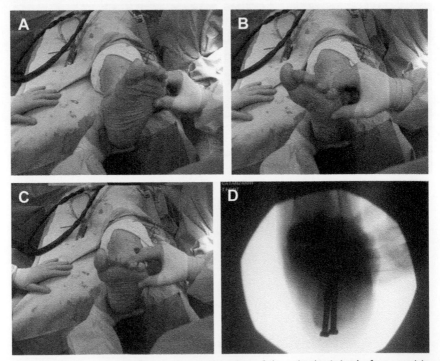

Fig. 18. (*A*) Maximum pronation during positioning of the subtalar joint before provisional fixation. (*B*) Maximum supination. (*C*) Neutral position. (*D*) Axial image showing relationship of the calcaneus to the tibia.

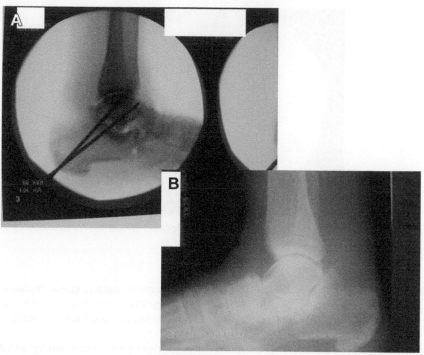

Fig. 19. (*A*) Preoperative lateral view of stage 3 posterior tibial tendon dysfunction. (*B*) Intraoperative lateral image showing restoration of calcaneal inclination and provisional pin fixation.

into the talus. A helpful tip is to have the surgeon palpate the distal aspect of the anterior tibial crest with the fingers of his or her nondominant hand, aiming the guide wire toward this point of reference while confirming the wire's course with fluoroscopy on the lateral view (**Fig. 20**). A second guide pin should then be placed in a similar

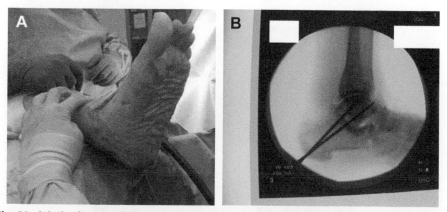

Fig. 20. (*A*) The fingers of the nondominant hand are placed along the distal aspect of the anterior tibial crest; this will serve as a target for placement of guide pins. (*B*) Lateral intraoperative image showing guide-pin placement.

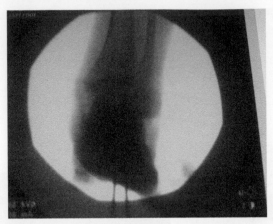

Fig. 21. AP image of the ankle showing guide pins located within the talus.

direction. An AP image of the ankle should be obtained before screw delivery to ensure that the pins do not invade the ankle joint (**Fig. 21**). Screw length is measured and confirmed on a lateral image. The large-diameter screws are then delivered over the guide pins (**Fig. 22**).

The TNJ is the second joint to be addressed. Realignment is obtained by adducting the forefoot on the hindfoot and rotating the medial column in a plantar direction. The forefoot should parallel the hindfoot in the frontal and transverse planes. An AP image should demonstrate the talar head to be completely covered by the navicular and the talus–first metatarsal angle reduced to zero. A lateral image should also show the talus–first metatarsal angle to be zero, indicating sagittal plane realignment. The authors typically use smaller-diameter screws in this joint. A guide pin is then inserted from the inferior aspect of the navicular tuberosity into the head and neck of the talus. This action is performed under image

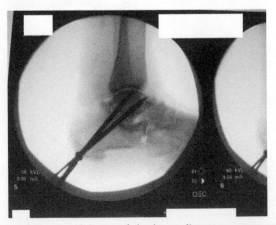

Fig. 22. Lateral image following delivery of the large-diameter screws over guide pins.

intensification on a lateral view, and an AP image should be obtained to confirm adequate placement within the talus (**Fig. 23**). A second pin is then placed from the dorsal aspect of the distal navicular into the midsubstance of the talus. This pin should be in the lateral aspect of the joint. This maneuver should be performed under lateral image intensification and then confirmed on an AP image. Measurements are then taken, and cannulated screws delivered over the guide pins (**Fig. 24**).

There is little positioning required for the calcaneocuboid joint, as its position has been secured by positioning and fixation of the STJ and TNJ. Fixation can be accomplished with 2 small-diameter cannulated screws placed in various constructs (**Fig. 25**). Alternatives include the use of 1 large-diameter screw in an axial fashion placed from either distal to proximal or proximal to distal, and staple fixation (**Fig. 26**).

Hemostasis and Closure

The pneumatic thigh tourniquet is released and hemostasis is achieved following osteosynthesis. Any small defects can then be packed with bone graft. The authors often decorticate the undersurface of the talus and dorsal aspect of the calcaneus. This area is then packed with a combination of bone graft and bone graft substitute that provides osteoinduction. A closed suction drain is placed and closure performed. A popliteal nerve block is performed to aid in postoperative pain management.

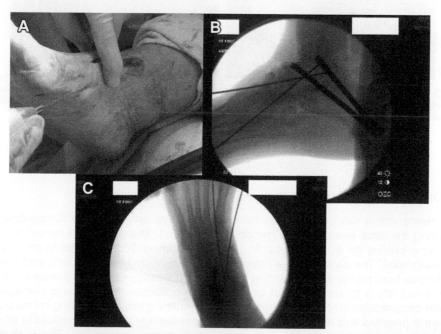

Fig. 23. (*A*) The initial guide pin for fixation of the talonavicular joint is delivered just inferior to the navicular tuberosity. (*B*) Lateral image confirming guide-pin placement. Note restoration of the talus–first metatarsal angle. (*C*) AP image confirming guide-pin placement. Note complete coverage of the talar head.

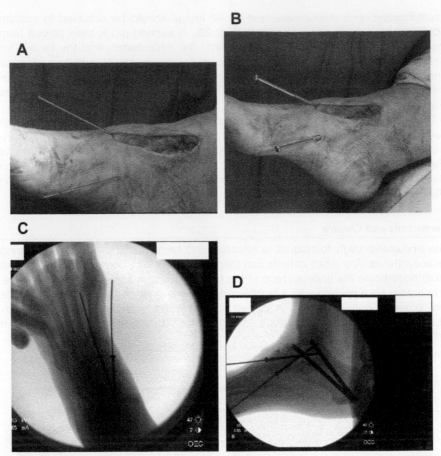

Fig. 24. (*A*) Intraoperative image showing guide-pin placement within the talonavicular joint. (*B*) Delivery of small-diameter screws over guide pins. (*C*) AP image following screw delivery. (*D*) Lateral image following screw delivery.

POSTOPERATIVE MANAGEMENT

Patients with a risk of deep vein thrombosis receive prophylactic anticoagulation during the initial postoperative immobilization period. The patient will remain non–weight bearing for 6 to 8 weeks or until osseous consolidation is noted on serial radiographs. The patient is then transitioned to a walking fracture boot, and progresses from partial weight bearing to full weight bearing over 2 to 3 weeks, with eventual return to standard foot gear. Residual postoperative edema is managed with compression stockings on transition to the walking boot. Depending on the patient's progress and length of recovery, physical therapy may be beneficial in promoting a more comfortable and expeditious return to activity. The authors especially consider physical therapy if the posterior muscle group has been lengthened in an elderly person.

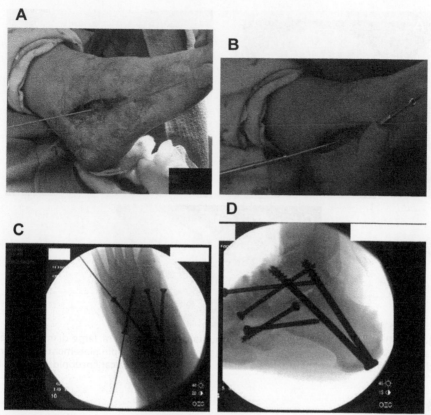

Fig. 25. (*A*) Intraoperative image showing guide-pin placement for calcaneocuboid joint. (*B*) Small-diameter screw delivery over guide pins. (*C*) AP radiograph confirming screw placement. (*D*) Lateral image confirming small-diameter screw placement.

COMPLICATIONS

Complications following triple arthrodesis include nonunion, malunion/malposition, anterior or lateral impingement, fixation problems, loss of correction, and progressive degenerative joint disease of the ankle. The incidence of nonunion following triple arthrodesis for adult acquired flatfoot is relatively low in comparison with those patients undergoing triple arthrodesis for posttraumatic arthritis. Adequate joint preparation, 2-point fixation, and adequate non–weight bearing until consolidation are important factors related to prevention of nonunion. Unfortunately, nonunion is often associated with malunion, and this requires revisional surgery. Malposition can be avoided by meticulous intraoperative positioning, using both clinical and radiographic confirmation. Lateral impingement is often the result of inadequate realignment of a severe valgus deformity. Anterior impingement is secondary to overcorrection when reducing the talonavicular joint, which can result in a horizontal talus and subsequent decrease in range of motion of the ankle joint. Ankle joint arthritis is not uncommon following triple arthrodesis. However, most ankle arthritis is asymptomatic. Pell and

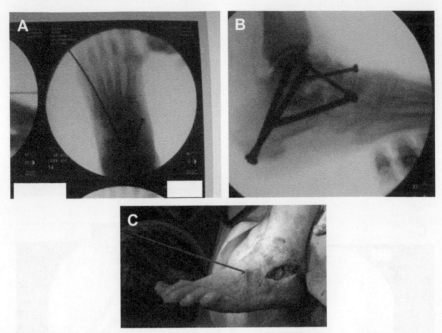

Fig. 26. (*A*) Intraoperative image showing guide-pin placement of large-diameter screw fixating the calcaneocuboid joint. (*B*) AP image confirming guide-pin placement. (*C*) Lateral radiograph showing axial-placed large-diameter screw for the calcaneocuboid joint.

colleagues[7] demonstrated that patient satisfaction did not correlate with the degree of deformity or ankle arthritis following triple arthrodesis. Rather, patient satisfaction correlated with postoperative alignment.

SUMMARY

Triple arthrodesis for adult acquired flatfoot results in universally good outcomes. Patients typically demonstrate decreased symptoms and an improved level of function. This procedure has been proved to be reasonably predictable. Results are enhanced with adequate preparation of joint surfaces, bone graft/bone graft substitutes, 2-point fixation of all tritarsal joints, a vertical heel position, and extra-articular arthrodesis. Adequate realignment is the most critical factor related to outcome.

REFERENCES

1. Fortin PT, Walling AK. Triple arthrodesis. Clin Orthop Relat Res 1999;(365):91–9.
2. Bennett GL, Graham CE, Mauldin DM. Triple arthrodesis in adults. Foot Ankle 1991;12:138–43.
3. Bednarz PA, Monroe MT, Manoli A. Triple arthrodesis in adults. Foot Ankle Int 1999;20:356–63.
4. Catanzariti AR, Mendicino RW, Maskill MP. Posterior tibial tendon dysfunction. In: Southerland JT, editor. McGlamry's comprehensive textbook of foot and ankle surgery, vol. 1, 4th edition. Philadelphia: Lippincott Williams & Wilkins; 2012. p. 636–69.

5. Resnick RB, Jahss MH, Choueka J, et al. Deltoid ligament forces after tibialis posterior tendon rupture: effects of triple arthrodesis and calcaneal displacement osteotomies. Foot Ankle Int 1995;16(5):314.
6. Song SJ, Lee S, O'Malley MJ, et al. Deltoid ligament strain after correction of acquired flatfoot deformity by triple arthrodesis. Foot Ankle Int 2000;21(7):573–7.
7. Pell RF, Myerson MS, Schon LC. Clinical outcome after primary triple arthrodesis. J Bone Joint Surg Am 2000;82(1):47–57.

Double Arthrodesis Through a Medial Approach for End-Stage Adult-Acquired Flatfoot

Alan R. Catanzariti, DPM*, Adebola T. Adeleke, DPM

KEYWORDS

- Double arthrodesis • Medial approach • End-stage adult-acquired flatfoot

KEY POINTS

- Selective arthrodesis of the talonavicular and subtalar joints (double arthrodesis) for end-stage adult-acquired flatfoot is a reasonable alternative to triple arthrodesis when the lateral skin is deficient or transverse plane subluxation is pronounced.
- Advantages of selective talonavicular and subtalar joint arthrodesis include reduction in lateral wound complications, decreased incidence of nonunion, improved intraoperative visualization, and shorter operative times.
- Although double arthrodesis is recommended for stage III and stage IV adult-acquired flatfoot, triple arthrodesis is ideal for the most severe, nonreducible deformities.

INTRODUCTION

Triple arthrodesis has traditionally been the procedure of choice for end-stage adult-acquired flatfoot. The results have been universally good, with relatively high patient satisfaction. Furthermore, triple arthrodesis has proven to be a dependable and predictable procedure. Nonetheless, complications have been reported following triple arthrodesis in certain groups of patients. These complications include an increased risk of degeneration in surrounding joints, inadequate realignment when severe transverse plane deformity exists, increased risk of a residual supinatus/varus deformity in patients with severe peritalar subluxation, and lateral wound problems in patients with a combination of severe valgus deformity and deficient lateral skin.[1–6] Additionally, the calcaneocuboid joint (CCJ) may require bone grafting following realignment of a severe deformity.[7]

Disclosure: Author has nothing to disclose.

Division of Foot & Ankle Surgery, West Penn Hospital, 4800 Friendship Avenue, N1, Pittsburgh, PA 15224, USA

* Corresponding author. 4955 Steubenville Pike, Suite 189, Pittsburgh, PA 15205.

E-mail address: acatanzariti@faiwp.com

Clin Podiatr Med Surg 31 (2014) 435–444

http://dx.doi.org/10.1016/j.cpm.2014.04.001
podiatric.theclinics.com

Selective arthrodesis of the talonavicular joint (TNJ) and subtalar joint (STJ) through a single medial approach has been developed as an alternative surgical option to help avoid or diminish the incidence of complications sometimes encountered with triple arthrodesis.[8–16] Indications for this procedure include end-stage adult-acquired flatfoot (stage III or IV) when deformity is usually severe and nonreducible. The authors especially prefer this procedure with severe transverse plane deformity, where an Anteroposterior (AP) radiograph demonstrates severe subluxation or dislocation of the TNJ. This procedure is also ideal in those patients with a combination of severe deformity and deficient lateral skin that might predispose them to lateral wound dehiscence following realignment. The authors often choose this approach as an alternative to triple arthrodesis in high-risk patients, including those patients with diabetes mellitus, rheumatoid arthritis, long-term steroid use, and the elderly.

TECHNIQUE

The procedure is performed through medial incision beginning just posterior to the medial malleolus and extending to the medial cuneiform. The authors sometimes carry the incision further distally if a naviculocuneiform or first tarsometatarsal arthrodesis is part of the reconstruction. A full-thickness incision is made just dorsal to the posterior tibial tendon. The tendon is inspected, and if severe tendinosis is noted, the entire tendon is evacuated. If, however, the tendon appears to be viable and healthy, the tendon is preserved. A complete release of all periarticular structures about the TNJ and STJ, including the interosseous and bifurcate ligaments, is essential. This permits adequate intra-articular visualization for cartilage debridement and joint preparation. Additionally, thorough release of contracted soft tissue structures allows easier reduction of the deformity. However, caution should be exercised during proximal dissection about the malleolus with care taken to avoid excess transection of the anterior portion of the deltoid ligament. Overzealous transaction of the anterior portion of deltoid ligament might predispose the ankle to valgus deformity, especially if hindfoot realignment is not adequate. Furthermore, the authors typically identify the flexor hallucis longus tendon, and sometimes, the flexor digitorum longus tendon, and protect them throughout the case. A combination of lamina spreaders and pin distractors can then be utilized to provide access to the STJ. Sharp, curved osteotomes and currettes are used to debride the cartilage. Angled Currettes are ideal for debriding cartilage from the posterior facet. After the distractors have been present for a period of time, and the cartilage has been debrided from the posterior facet, the posterior-lateral joint capsule is visible (**Fig. 1**). The authors carefully release this structure. All debris is then evacuated from the STJ prior to joint preparation. This includes soft tissue structures distal to the articular surfaces, as the authors will prepare this area for arthrodesis to extend the fusion mass into the extra-articular area. The TNJ is then distracted for cartilage debridement and joint preparation in the same manner. Following lavage of both joints, the subchondral plates are fenestrated and weakened with a 2.5 mm drill and then methodically broken with a small osteotome (**Fig. 2**). The authors often augment these sites with demineralized bone matrix gel. The STJ is reduced into a neutral position, and the TNJ is then realigned and provisionally fixated with guide pins from a 4.5 mm cannulated screw system. This maneuver is performed under image intensification, checking AP, lateral, and axial images. The authors typically deliver the first screw medially, from the navicular tuberosity, to support realignment. The second screw is delivered percutaneously along the most lateral aspect of the TNJ. A third screw is sometimes delivered centrally. It is important to have even compression across the entire TNJ. The STJ is then fixated with 2 large-diameter

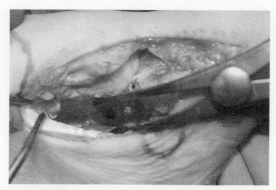

Fig. 1. Intraoperative inspection of the subtalar joint following debridement of the cartilage. The lateral capsule can be visualized.

cannulated screws delivered from inferior to superior (**Fig. 3**). The authors then perform a valgus stress test of the ankle under image intensification and proceed to repair the deltoid ligament if valgus is found. The wound is then closed in standard fashion over a closed suction drain. Patients are placed into a nonweight-bearing short-leg cast for 6 to 8 weeks, followed by a fracture boot for an additional 3 to 4 weeks. Postoperative decisions are based on serial radiographs and clinical findings such as edema and warmth.

ANCILLARY PROCEDURES

There are several ancillary procedures that are sometimes necessary in order to obtain a stable, plantigrade foot. Posterior muscle group lengthening, either in the

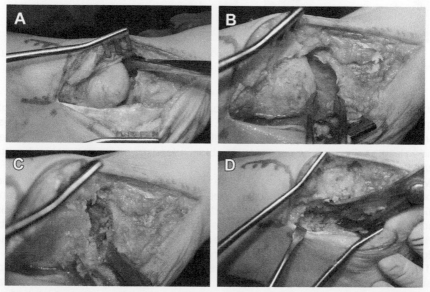

Fig. 2. (*A*) Exposure of the talonavicular joint. (*B*) Following debridement of articular cartilage. (*C, D*) Preparation of subchondral plates.

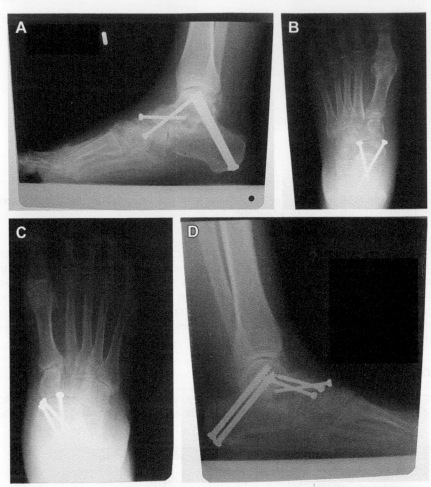

Fig. 3. (*A, B*) AP and lateral radiographs demonstrating standard fixation construct. (*C, D*) Three-screw construct for the talonavicular joint.

form of an Achilles tendon lengthening or gastrocnemius recession, is invariably required in stage III adult-acquired flatfoot. The authors utilize gastrocnemius recession in most cases. However, following realignment of a severe deformity, an Achilles tendon lengthening may be necessary to obtain adequate length and restore sagittal plane position.

Medial displacement osteotomy of the calcaneus can be used as an adjunct procedure to address ankle valgus or medial soft tissue attenuation. Resnick and colleagues[17] have shown that a triple arthrodesis, in combination with a medial displacement osteotomy of the calcaneus, will reduce deltoid ligament forces by 56%. Song and colleagues[18] have also suggested that medializing the calcaneus following triple arthrodesis would protect the deltoid complex (**Fig. 4**).

The authors will consider medial column stabilization, either in the form of naviculo-cuneiform arthrodesis or first tarsometatarsal arthrodesis, when medial column instability is identified following triple arthrodesis for stage III adult-acquired flatfoot. Insufficiency of the medial column can result in a functional varus. Failure to address

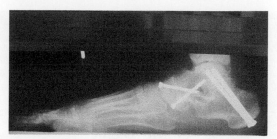

Fig. 4. Addition of medial displacement osteotomy of the calcaneus.

medial column instability can result in a lateral column overload when patients begin weight bearing (**Fig. 5**).

Harvesting of regional bone graft and/or bone marrow aspirate is a part of virtually every hindfoot arthrodesis. Cancellous bone is often harvested from the calcaneus, utilizing 6 to 8 mm trephines through small lateral incisions. Bone marrow aspirate is obtained from the calcaneus prior to tourniquet inflation. The cancellous bone is packed into arthrodesis sites. The extra-articular areas along the under surface of the talus and the dorsal surface of the calcaneus are decorticated. The bone marrow aspirate is mixed with bioactive glass and then packed into this extra-articular area (**Fig. 6**).

Transfer of peroneus brevis to peroneus longest tendon is performed when the deformity is rather severe. Severe contracture of the peroneus brevis tendon can sometimes make it difficult to obtain complete realignment. As an alternative, the authors sometime transect both tendons.

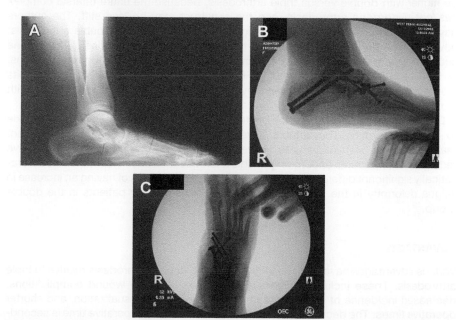

Fig. 5. (*A–C*) Radiographs demonstrating the addition of naviculocuneiform osteotomy to address medial column instability.

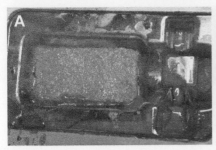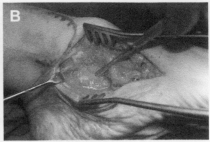

Fig. 6. (*A*, *B*) Bone marrow aspirate combined with bioactive glass is packed into the extra-articular sites to enhance arthrodesis and increase the fusion mass.

POTENTIAL PROBLEMS

Inadequate realignment of a severe deformity following double arthrodesis through a medial approach can occur. This is always a possibility without the release of severely contracted lateral soft tissue structures. The authors try to perform an intra-articular release of the lateral STJ capsule when possible. In situations in which adequate realignment is not possible following thorough release of soft tissue structures, the authors will consider osseous decompression through the TNJ. A sagittal saw is used to debride the joint until realignment is obtained in both transverse sagittal planes (**Fig. 7**). The authors also consider a medial displacement osteotomy of the calcaneus as an ancillary procedure if there is residual deformity following provisional fixation of the arthrodesis.

Nonunion is also a potential problem. Theoretically, the incidence of nonunion might be higher with double versus triple arthrodesis, because the entire tritarsal complex has not undergone arthrodesis, and the construct may be less stiff. The authors have encountered a number of nonunions of the TNJ following double arthrodesis; however, they do not have a statistical comparison to triple arthrodesis (**Fig. 8**). One such study is currently underway (Glenn Weinraub, DPM, personal communications, 2014). The authors have changed their fixation construct to include 3 screws across the talonavicular joint. Additionally, they sometimes supplement screw fixation with a medial locking plate.

Dissection of the anterior portion of the deltoid ligament might predispose the ankle to valgus deformity. The authors have encountered this situation when hindfoot realignment has been inadequate. However, 1 recent study comparing postoperative radiographs in patients undergoing double and triple arthrodesis demonstrated a statistically significant difference between the 2 groups. The odds of having an increase in valgus deformity in the triple group was 3.64 times that for patients in the double group.[19]

ADVANTAGES

Various advantages have been described for using double arthrodesis relative to triple arthrodesis. These include a significant reduction in lateral wound complications, decreased incidence of nonunion, improved intraoperative visualization, and shorter operative times. The decreased risk of nonunion and shorter operative time is secondary to sparing the CCJ. Transverse plane realignment of a severely abducted foot might be easier if the lateral column is not shortened by CCJ arthrodesis. One study

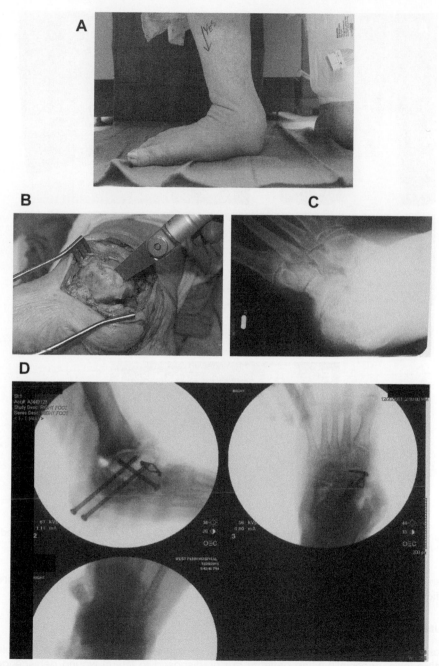

Fig. 7. (*A, B*) Severe deformity being treated with decompression of the talonavicular joint. (*C, D*) Preoperative AP radiograph and intraoperative realignment.

observed that distraction of the CCJ may reduce the risk of degenerative joint disease at this site.[15] Other studies describe the protective effect of motion remaining at the CCJ following double arthrodesis and the decreased incidence of arthritis on surrounding joints compared with triple arthrodesis.[8,14,20] Another recent study

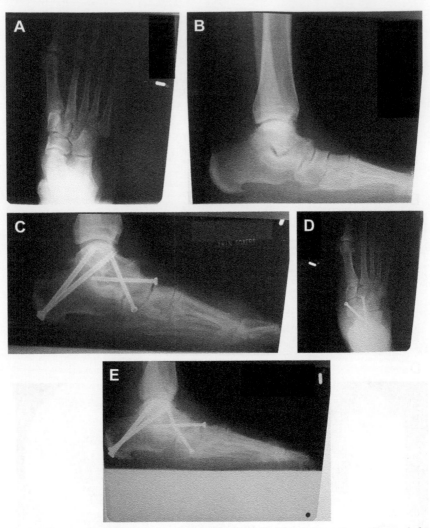

Fig. 8. (*A*, *B*) AP and lateral preoperative radiographs. (*C*, *D*) Postoperative radiograph feed. (*E*) Nonunion of the talonavicular joint.

demonstrated that double arthrodesis through a medial approach was both more efficient and cost-effective than traditional triple arthrodesis.[21]

SUMMARY

Double arthrodesis through a medial approach is a reasonable alternative to triple arthrodesis, especially when patients are predisposed to lateral wound dehiscence secondary to a severe deformity, deficient lateral skin, or have risk factors that adversely affect their wound healing potential. Most research evaluating this procedure has been level IV. A recent review on a series of 18 feet undergoing single-incision medial approach double arthrodesis for posterior tibial tendon dysfunction reported a union rate of 89%, with 2 malunions and 2 valgus ankles. There were no wound complications, and the satisfaction rate was 78%. However, the results were not encouraging enough for the authors to recommend adopting this approach as an alternative to triple arthrodesis.[22] Although the authors prefer double arthrodesis for stage III and IV Adult Acquired Flatfoot (AAFF), they continue to employ triple arthrodesis for the most severe, nonreducible deformities. Although radiographic improvement is acceptable and predictable following double arthrodesis, the authors have found that the clinical appearance is not as good as patients undergoing triple arthrodesis. A prospective, randomized study comparing double with triple arthrodesis for surgical management of stage III adult-acquired flatfoot would be beneficial. This type of study might help identify which deformities are best treated by either double or triple arthrodesis.

REFERENCES

1. Graves SC, Mann RA, Graves KO. Triple arthrodesis in older adults: results after long-term follow-up. J Bone Joint Surg Am 1993;75:355–62.
2. Figgie MP, O'Malley MJ, Ranawat C, et al. Triple arthrodesis in rheumatoid arthritis. Clin Orthop Relat Res 1993;(292):250–4.
3. Salzman CL, Fehrle MJ, Copper RR, et al. Triple arthrodesis: twenty five and forty four year average follow-up of the same patients. J Bone Joint Surg Am 1999;81: 1391–402.
4. Pell RF, Myerson MS, Schon LC. Clinical outcome after primary triple arthrodesis. J Bone Joint Surg Am 2000;82:47–57.
5. Knupp M, Skoog A, Tornkvist H, et al. Triple arthrodesis in rheumatoid arthritis: a retrospective long-term study of 32 cases. Foot Ankle Int 2008,29:293–7.
6. Rosenfeld PF, Budgen SA, Saxby TS. Triple arthrodesis is bone grafting necessary?: the results in 100 consecutive cases. J Bone Joint Surg Br 2005;87: 175–8.
7. Lee MS. Medial approach to the severe valgus foot. Clin Podiatr Med Surg 2007; 24:735–44.
8. Jeng CL, Vora AM, Myerson MS. The medial approach to triple arthrodesis: indications and technique for management of rigid valgus deformities in high-risk patients. Foot Ankle Clin 2005;10:515–21.
9. Vora AM, Myerson MS, Jeng CL. The medial approach to triple arthrodesis: indications and technique for management of rigid valgus deformities in high-risk patients. Tech Foot Ankle Surg 2005;4(4):258–62.
10. O'Malley MJ, Deland JT, Lee KT. Selective hindfoot arthrodesis for the treatment of adult acquired flatfoot deformity: an in vitro study. Foot Ankle Int 1995;16: 411–7.
11. Brillhault J. Single medial approach to modified double arthrodesis in rigid flatfoot with lateral deficient skin. Foot Ankle Int 2009;30(1):21–6.
12. Sammarco VJ, Magur EG, Sammarco GJ, et al. Arthrodesis of the subtalar and talonavicular joints for correction of symptomatic hindfoot malalignment. Foot Ankle Int 2006;27(9):661–6.
13. Jeng CL, Tankson CJ, Myerson MS. The single medial approach to triple arthrodesis: a cadaver study. Foot Ankle Int 2006;27:1122–5.
14. Jackson WF, Tryfonidis M, Cooke PH, et al. Arthrodesis of the hindfoot for valgus deformity: an entirely medial approach. J Bone Joint Surg Br 2007;89:925–7.
15. Knupp M, Schuh R, Stufkens SA, et al. Subtalar and talonavicular arthrodesis through a single medial approach for the correction of severe planovalgus deformity. J Bone Joint Surg Br 2009;91:612–5.
16. Weinraib GM, Schuberth JM, Lee M, et al. Isolated medial incisional approach to subtalar and talonavicular arthrodesis. J Foot Ankle Surg 2010;49:326–30.

17. Resnick RB, Jahss MH, Choueka J, et al. Deltoid ligament forces after tibialis posterior tendon rupture: effects of triple arthrodesis and calcaneal displacement osteotomies. Foot Ankle Int 1995;16(1):14–20.
18. Song SJ, Lee S, O'Malley MJ, et al. Deltoid ligament strain after correction of acquired flatfoot deformity by triple arthrodesis. Foot Ankle Int 2000;21(7):573–7.
19. Hyer CF, Galli MM, Scott RT, et al. Ankle valgus after hindfoot arthrodesis: a radiographic and chart comparison of the medial double and triple arthrodeses. J Foot Ankle Surg 2014;53(1):55–8.
20. Gelleman H, Lenihan M, Halikis N, et al. Selective tarsal arthrodesis: an in vitro analysis of the effect on foot motion. Foot Ankle 1987;8:127–33.
21. Galli MM, Scott RT, Bussewitz BW, et al. A retrospective comparison of cost and efficiency of the medial double and dual incision triple arthrodeses. Foot Ankle Spec 2014;7(1):32–6.
22. Anand P, Nunley JA, DeOrio JK. Single-incision medial approach for double arthrodesis of hindfoot in posterior tibialis tendon dysfunction. Foot Ankle Int 2013;34(3):338–44.

Surgical Decision Making for Stage IV Adult Acquired Flatfoot Disorder

Kyle S. Peterson, DPM, AACFAS*, Christopher F. Hyer, DPM, MS

KEYWORDS

- Posterior tibial tendon dysfunction • Adult acquired flatfoot deformity • Ankle valgus
- Deltoid ligament insufficiency • Deltoid ligament reconstruction

KEY POINTS

- Stage IV adult acquired flatfoot disorder is characterized by tibiotalar ankle valgus tilting within the mortise.
- Stage IV flatfoot deformity is subclassified into stage IV-A, flexible ankle valgus without significant arthritis, and stage IV-B, rigid ankle valgus with significant arthritis.
- Stage IV-A surgical treatment is centered on reconstruction of the failed deltoid ligament.
- Stage IV-B surgical treatment focuses on realignment of the deformity with tibiotalocalcaneal or pantalar arthrodesis.

INTRODUCTION

Adult acquired flatfoot deformity (AAFD) is a debilitating musculoskeletal condition affecting the lower extremity. Posterior tibial tendon dysfunction (PTTD) is the primary etiology for the development of a flatfoot deformity in an adult.[1] In 1989, Johnson and Strom created the most utilized classification for PTTD.[2] Stage I PTTD is characterized by pain and edema along the medial aspect of the hindfoot and involves posterior tibial tendon tendonitis without associated hindfoot deformity. Stage II PTTD is depicted by a flexible flatfoot deformity with hindfoot valgus, forefoot abduction, and forefoot varus. Stage III PTTD is a more advanced disease causing a fixed, rigid hindfoot deformity. In 1996, Myerson modified the 3 stages of PTTD by adding a fourth stage involving the ankle joint.[3,4] Stage IV PTTD occurs when the talus tilts into a valgus position within the ankle mortise (**Fig. 1**). This is caused primarily by insufficiency of

Advanced Foot and Ankle Surgical Fellowship, Orthopedic Foot and Ankle Center, 300 Polaris Parkway, Suite 2000, Westerville, OH 43082, USA
* Corresponding author. Attn: Research, Orthopedic Foot & Ankle Center, 300 Polaris Parkway, Suite 2000, Westerville, OH 43082.
E-mail address: ofacresearch@orthofootankle.com

Clin Podiatr Med Surg 31 (2014) 445–454
http://dx.doi.org/10.1016/j.cpm.2014.03.001
0891-8422/14/$ – see front matter © 2014 Elsevier Inc. All rights reserved.

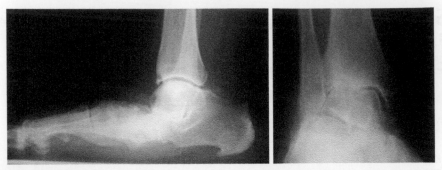

Fig. 1. Lateral foot and anteroposterior ankle radiographs demonstrating stage IV AAFD. Severe pes planus foot deformity is seen in conjunction with tibiotalar valgus angulation.

the deltoid ligament.[5] Recently, stage IV PTTD has been subdivided into stage IV-A and IV-B.[6] Stage IV-A classifies patients with hindfoot valgus and a flexible ankle valgus without significant tibiotalar arthritis, while stage IV-B involves a rigid ankle valgus with significant tibiotalar arthritis.[6]

ANATOMIC CONSIDERATIONS

Although the posterior tibial tendon (PTT) is the primary dynamic stabilizer on the medial arch, other anatomic structures contribute to the deforming forces on the hindfoot and midfoot. As the PTT assumes greater dysfunction and tendinosis, the peroneus brevis begins to act as an unopposed muscle, leading to increased hindfoot eversion. A contracted gastrocnemius–soleus muscle complex also leads to increased hindfoot eversion. Additional static ligamentous structures on the medial foot and ankle also contribute to the loss of the medial longitudinal arch, including the spring ligament complex, interosseous talocalcaneal, and the superficial deltoid ligament.[7,8]

The deltoid ligament consists of both superficial and deep fibers. The superficial band is a wide, fan-shaped portion that extends from the navicular to the posterior tibiotalar capsule and is incorporated into the superiomedial portion of the spring ligament.[6] The deep portion of the deltoid ligament originates from the intercollicular groove and the posterior colliculus of the medial malleolus and inserts of the medial aspect of the talar body.[9] Generally, the superficial deltoid is comprised of the tibionavicular, tibiocalcaneal, and tibiotalar ligaments, while the deep is composed of the anterior and posterior tibiotalar ligaments.[9]

Contributions from both the superficial and deep components of the deltoid ligament resist against tibiotalar tilting.[10,11] Harper demonstrated in a cadaver study that division of both the superficial and deep components produced an average of 14° of valgus talar tilting.[11] Earll and colleagues,[10] in another cadaver study, showed a 20% to 30% increase in tibiotalar joint pressures and a 26% to 43% decrease in contact areas with sectioning of the tibiocalcaneal fibers of the superficial deltoid. Moreover, Rasmussen and colleagues[12–14] have performed multiple cadaveric sectioning studies demonstrating superficial deltoid fibers contributing to the primary restraint of ankle valgus angulation.

PATIENT EVALUATION

Patients with stage IV PTTD will typically present similar to those with a rigid stage III foot. Additionally, stage IV patients will complain of medial ankle pain, often with an advanced valgus foot deformity. A history of associated ankle weakness and swelling is common. Patients frequently present with a multitude of failed braces, orthotics, and shoes. In those patients with severe ankle valgus, lateral ankle pain may also cause pain and debilitation. As the ankle valgus becomes more of a fixed deformity, forces are transferred to the fibula, where a stress fracture is possible, termed Johnson stage V disease.[15] Patients are unable to perform single or double heel rise tests. The rigidity of the talonavicular and subtalar joints will be evident with manual range of motion. The ankle joint will be painful on palpation, and a determination of whether the ankle deformity is fixed or flexible should be noted. The gastrocnemius–soleus muscle complex and peroneal tendons will often be contracted.

Radiographic examination should include standing images of both the foot and ankle. Anteroposterior and lateral foot radiographs will demonstrate increased talo-first metatarsal angles, dorsolateral peritalar subluxation, loss of talar head coverage with the navicular, and decreased calcaneal inclination angle.

Weight-bearing anteroposterior and mortise ankle images will demonstrate increased tibiotalar valgus tilting with stage IV PTTD. In addition to the valgus tilt present in the ankle, the magnitude of tibiotalar arthritis should also be determined. When a valgus talar tilt is recognized in a patient with AAFD, the ability to passively correct the deformity needs to be tested. Evaluation is performed by manually applying a varus force of the joint under direct fluoroscopy (**Fig. 2**). If needed, contralateral comparison radiographs and stress fluoroscopic films may be necessary. Advanced imaging with magnetic resonance imaging (MRI) may be of benefit to evaluate the integrity of the posterior tibial tendon, deltoid ligament complex, and degeneration present in the ankle and hindfoot.

TREATMENT OF STAGE IV

Nonoperative management of AAFD relies on supporting the foot externally with braces or orthotics. Management of earlier stages is successful with rest, immobilization, anti-inflammatory medications, and physical therapy.[16] Stage IV AAFD, however, is difficult to treat conservatively, and treatment is often unsuccessful.[17] The standard University of California Biomechanics Laboratory inserts are usually ineffective at

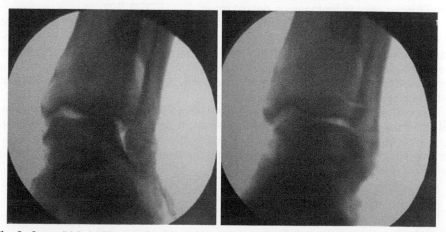

Fig. 2. Stage IV-A AAFD. A reducible ankle valgus without significant tibiotalar arthritis is seen here (*left*). A manual varus force is applied under direct fluoroscopy to determine reducibility (*right*).

controlling the rigid deformity of the foot and off-loading the ankle valgus. Custom molded ankle–foot orthoses and Arizona style braces can be of benefit in stage IV; however, pain and advancing tibiotalar arthritis may not be adequately corrected.

With conservative treatment oftentimes failing, surgical management is indicated frequently in stage IV patients. There is no gold standard on which to base surgical treatment for stage IV. Historically, tibiotalar valgus tilt with some extent of arthritis has been treated with a tibiotalar fusion.[15] The rigid flatfoot that remains, however, still needs to be treated, which leads to selective hindfoot fusions in addition to the tibiotalar fusion. This creates the standard tibiotalocalcaneal or traditional pantalar fusion for a patient with stage IV AAFD (**Fig. 3**).[5] These major hindfoot and ankle fusions have been successful in re-establishing alignment, but often create residual pain and stiffness.[18,19]

It is important to group patients into the subclassification for stage IV AAFD, IV-A (flexible ankle valgus without significant tibiotalar arthritis) or IV-B (rigid ankle valgus or flexible ankle valgus with significant tibiotalar arthritis).[5] This aids in determining the appropriate surgical indications for stage IV, with IV-A being treated with ankle joint-sparing procedures, and IV-B treated with ankle joint destructive procedures.

Ankle Joint-Sparing Surgery

Stage IV-A PTTD can be treated with procedures that correct the ankle valgus and flatfoot deformity while preserving motion in the ankle joint. One must be certain the ankle joint is flexible, without degeneration, in order to re-establish alignment. This reducibility maneuver can be performed by intra- or preoperative fluoroscopic examination (see **Fig. 2**).

Reconstruction of the deltoid ligament complex is the primary operation for realignment of tibiotalar valgus in stage IV.[5,6,15] A well-aligned reconstructed foot is imperative to the success of a concomitant deltoid ligament repair, and therefore, flatfoot reconstruction should be performed before repairing the deltoid complex. Hindfoot fusions, such as a triple or medial double arthrodesis should be performed prior to repair of the deltoid ligament in order to provide a stable plantigrade foot for proper ligamentous tensioning.[1,20] For the occasional flexible flatfoot with ankle valgus, reconstruction can be obtained with hindfoot and/or midfoot osteotomies rather than fusions prior to ligamentous deltoid repair.

Numerous reports of deltoid ligament repair have been reported and are divided into 3 classes: primary repair of the host tissue, advancement of host tissue, and reconstruction with autograft or allograft tissue.[6,21–26] Some of the earliest reports of primary repair and advancement and reefing of the native deltoid ligament tissue did provide a congruent tibiotalar joint, but ultimately failed because of the poor quality of tissue that was incompetent during stage IV disease.[6,26]

Autograft or allograft reconstruction of ankle valgus is now favored over direct repair of native tissue. The importance of strong healthy tissue to reconstruct both the deep and superficial components of the deltoid ligament complex is recognized as a superior construct.[6] Reconstruction of the deltoid ligament complex has been described with many variations:

- Peroneus longus autograft[22,23]
- Flexor hallucis longus autograft[15]
- Posterior tibial tendon autograft[27]
- Achilles tendon allograft[28]
- Forked hamstring allograft[6,25]
- Looped semitendinosis allograft[24]

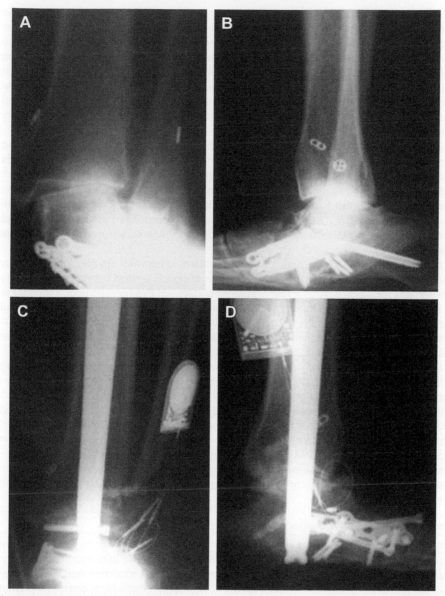

Fig. 3. (*A, B*) Stage IV-B AAFD. Failed triple and medial column arthrodesis with rigid ankle valgus and significant tibiotalar arthritis. (*C, D*) Pantalar arthrodesis with retrograde intramedullary nail and extended medial column fusion at the naviculocuneiform joint for stage IV-B AAFD.

The two most commonly utilized techniques have been described by Deland and colleagues[22] and Bluman and Myerson,[6] in which Deland described the use of peroneus longus autograft, and Bluman demonstrated a technique with forked hamstring allograft.[25] Deland, in 2004, reported on his autograft technique on 5 patients. The peroneus longus tendon was resected proximally and then passed from lateral to medial through a bony tunnel in the talus. A second bony tunnel was then made from the tip of the medial malleolus to the lateral distal third of the tibia, in which the graft was secured with suturing to a screw or a staple. The average talar tilt corrected was from 10° preoperative to 3.6° postoperative with a minimum 2-year follow-up. One patient was considered a failure with a residual 9° of talar tilt postoperatively. Ellis and colleagues[23] published a more recent follow-up of these same 5 patients in 2010. Intermediate follow-up at a mean 8.9 years revealed a mean talar tilt of 2° present postoperatively. Pitfalls of this technique involve reconstruction of only the deep deltoid component and not the superficial component, as well as donor site morbidity from the peroneus longus autograft.

In 2007, Bluman and Myerson described their technique with a forked hamstring allograft for reconstruction of both the superficial and deep deltoid complex.[6] This minimally invasive technique involves reconstruction with a 20 cm hamstring allograft split longitudinally, creating 2 limbs for insertion into the talus and calcaneus. The single limb is inserted into a tibial tunnel parallel to the ankle joint and fixated with an absorbable interference screw. The 2 limbs are then passed subcutaneously and fixated into the talus (recreated deep deltoid) and calcaneus (recreating superficial deltoid) with interference screws.

In 2011, Jeng and colleagues[25] reported patient outcomes utilizing this minimally invasive deltoid reconstruction technique with allograft tendon combined with triple arthrodesis for stage IV AAFD. Eight patients underwent this reconstruction technique at a mean follow-up of 36 months. Five of 8 patients were judged to have a successful outcome (valgus talar tilt <2°), with a reduction of tibiotalar valgus tilt from a mean 6.4° preoperative to 2.0° postoperative. The authors stated that patients with a tibiotalar valgus greater than 10° preoperative had poorer outcomes.

Haddad and colleagues[24] also recently described a technique in cadavers using anterior tibial tendon allograft recreating both the superficial and deep deltoid ligament. Endobuttons are used to secure the graft in tunnels in both the talus and calcaneus, while the residual graft is looped and passed through a tibia tunnel and fixated on the anterolateral tibia cortex with a cancellous screw and spiked washer. This reconstruction technique has been able to restore eversion and external rotation stability of the talus under low torque. Although tested with anterior tibial tendon allograft, the authors have now switched to using a cadaveric semitendinous tendon to decrease bulkiness. No study has been published regarding clinical outcomes with this technique.

Ankle Joint Destructive Surgery

Stage IV-B AAFD, rigid ankle valgus deformity or flexible ankle valgus with significant tibiotalar arthritis does not lend itself to reconstructive deltoid ligament surgery. Rather, successful realignment of the ankle and hindfoot is accomplished with tibiotalocalcaneal or pantalar fusions (see **Fig. 3**).[5,15] Although reliable in reconstructing large and painful deformities, studies have shown residual pain, higher risk of nonunion, increased energy expenditure, and decreased functional capacity with tibiotalocalcaneal and pantalar fusion.[18,19,29]

If patients have a desire to preserve motion in the ankle joint, a treatment option to consider for stage IV-B AAFD is realignment of the flatfoot with hindfoot fusions or osteotomies combined with total ankle arthroplasty.[15] According to Bohay and Anderson, a type of stage IV AAFD patient with a relatively flexible flatfoot may be treated with conventional osteotomy or hindfoot fusion methods with an additional total ankle arthroplasty.[15] Other authors have also proposed subtalar or triple arthrodesis combined with a total ankle arthroplasty, although limited data have been published on patient outcomes with these methods.[30,31]

Additionally, reconstruction of the deltoid ligament complex combined with a total ankle arthroplasty is another alternative treatment option to avoid a large hindfoot and ankle fusion.[5,30,31] If a patient has had a previously failed deltoid ligament reconstruction, total ankle arthroplasty is generally not recommended. However, if the foot is balanced, and the deltoid ligament is attenuated, but not failed, a deltoid reconstruction procedure and total ankle arthroplasty may be combined. More research is needed to determine the long-term results of combined deltoid ligament reconstruction with total ankle arthroplasty.

ANKLE VALGUS AFTER HINDFOOT ARTHRODESIS

Although a triple or medial double arthrodesis has been considered the gold standard for treatment of stage III AAFD, postoperative ankle valgus remains a possibility (**Fig. 4**).[20,32–35] Malunion of a valgus hindfoot is one of the largest factors contributing to ankle valgus following a triple arthrodesis.[15] In a medial double arthrodesis, excessive surgical disruption of the deltoid ligament can weaken the structures and create a destabilized ankle, leading to a valgus deformity. Resnick and colleagues[36] demonstrated that a triple arthrodesis fused in a valgus or in situ position will lead to a 76% increase in deltoid ligament strain. The senior author most recently demonstrated a greater frequency of ankle valgus following triple arthrodesis compared with a medial double arthrodesis in 78 feet.[37] The odds of having an increase in ankle valgus following a triple arthrodesis was 3.64 times greater compared with patients in the medial double arthrodesis group for this comparative study. If postoperative ankle valgus is encountered following a hindfoot arthrodesis, reconstruction of the deltoid ligament may be performed if little tibiotalar arthritis is present. If a significant amount of tibiotalar arthritis is present with a larger valgus deformity, tibiotalar arthrodesis or

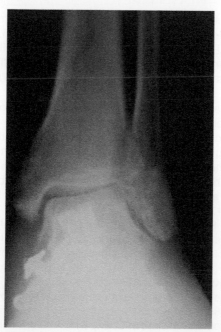

Fig. 4. Postoperative ankle valgus encountered following triple arthrodesis.

total ankle arthroplasty may be warranted. Further research is needed to examine postoperative ankle valgus following hindfoot arthrodesis and treatment options.

SUMMARY

Stage IV AAFD is difficult to surgically manage compared with earlier flatfoot stages. Dysfunction of the posterior tibial tendon with a decreased longitudinal arch and a valgus hindfoot is combined with valgus talar tilting within the ankle mortise. Insufficiency of the deltoid ligament is central in the pathoanatomy of this advanced stage of AAFD. Untreated, stage IV AAFD can lead to severe disability of the lower extremity. External bracing and orthoses may be initially utilized for conservative treatment; however, progression of the disorder often leads to surgical reconstruction. Stage IV-A is treated surgically with ankle joint-sparing procedures aimed at reconstructing the deltoid ligament complex with realignment of the valgus foot. Advanced degeneration found in stage IV-B often lends itself to ankle joint-destructive procedures, such as a tibiotalocalcaneal or pantalar arthrodesis, or, if possible, total ankle arthroplasty with a combined deltoid ligament reconstruction. With all procedures currently documented for stage IV AAFD, it is prudent to realign the ankle joint within the mortise, as well as the hindfoot under the leg, creating a stable plantigrade foot.

REFERENCES

1. Lee MS, Vanore JV, Thomas JL, et al. Diagnosis and treatment of adult flatfoot. J Foot Ankle Surg 2005;44:78–113.
2. Johnson KA, Strom DE. Tibialis posterior tendon dysfunction. Clin Orthop Relat Res 1989;(239):196–206.
3. Myerson M. Adult acquired flatfoot deformity. J Bone Joint Surg Am 1996;78: 780–92.
4. Myerson MS. Adult acquired flatfoot deformity: treatment of dysfunction of the posterior tibial tendon. Instr Course Lect 1997;46:393–405.
5. Smith JT, Bluman EM. Update on stage IV acquired adult flatfoot disorder: when the deltoid ligament becomes dysfunctional. Foot Ankle Clin 2012;17:351–60.
6. Bluman EM, Myerson MS. Stage IV posterior tibial tendon rupture. Foot Ankle Clin 2007;12:341–62.
7. Deland JT, De Asla RJ, Sung IH, et al. Posterior tibial tendon insufficiency: which ligaments are involved? Foot Ankle Int 2005;26:427–35.
8. Gazdag AR, Cracchiolo A 3rd. Rupture of the posterior tibial tendon. Evaluation of injury of the spring ligament and clinical assessment of tendon transfer and ligament repair. J Bone Joint Surg Am 1997;79:675–81.
9. Pankovich AM, Shivaram MS. Anatomical basis of variability in injuries of the medial malleolus and the deltoid ligament. I. Anatomical studies. Acta Orthop Scand 1979;50:217–23.
10. Earll M, Wayne J, Brodrick C, et al. Contribution of the deltoid ligament to ankle joint contact characteristics: a cadaver study. Foot Ankle Int 1996;17:317–24.
11. Harper MC. Deltoid ligament: an anatomical evaluation of function. Foot Ankle 1987;8:19–22.
12. Rasmussen O, Kromann-Andersen C, Boe S. Deltoid ligament. Functional analysis of the medial collateral ligamentous apparatus of the ankle joint. Acta Orthop Scand 1983;54:36–44.
13. Rasmussen O, Kromann-Andersen C. Experimental ankle injuries. Analysis of the traumatology of the ankle ligaments. Acta Orthop Scand 1983;54:356–62.

14. Rasmussen O. Stability of the ankle joint. Analysis of the function and traumatology of the ankle ligaments. Acta Orthop Scand Suppl 1985;211:1–75.
15. Bohay DR, Anderson JG. Stage iv posterior tibial tendon insufficiency: the tilted ankle. Foot Ankle Clin 2003;8:619–36.
16. Alvarez RG, Marini A, Schmitt C, et al. Stage I and II posterior tibial tendon dysfunction treated by a structured nonoperative management protocol: an orthosis and exercise program. Foot Ankle Int 2006;27:2–8.
17. Kelly IP, Nunley JA. Treatment of stage 4 adult acquired flatfoot. Foot Ankle Clin 2001;6:167–78.
18. Barrett GR, Meyer LC, Bray EW 3rd, et al. Pantalar arthrodesis: a long-term follow-up. Foot Ankle 1981;1:279–83.
19. Chou LB, Mann RA, Yaszay B, et al. Tibiotalocalcaneal arthrodesis. Foot Ankle Int 2000;21:804–8.
20. Weinraub GM, Schuberth JM, Lee M, et al. Isolated medial incisional approach to subtalar and talonavicular arthrodesis. J Foot Ankle Surg 2010; 49:326–30.
21. Boyer MI, Bowen V, Weiler P. Reconstruction of a severe grinding injury to the medial malleolus and the deltoid ligament of the ankle using a free plantaris tendon graft and vascularized gracilis free muscle transfer: case report. J Trauma 1994;36:454–7.
22. Deland JT, De Asla RJ, Segal A. Reconstruction of the chronically failed deltoid ligament: a new technique. Foot Ankle Int 2004;25:795–9.
23. Ellis SJ, Williams BR, Wagshul AD, et al. Deltoid ligament reconstruction with peroneus longus autograft in flatfoot deformity. Foot Ankle Int 2010;31: 781–9.
24. Haddad SL, Dedhia S, Ren Y, et al. Deltoid ligament reconstruction: a novel technique with biomechanical analysis. Foot Ankle Int 2010;31:639–51.
25. Jeng CL, Bluman EM, Myerson MS. Minimally invasive deltoid ligament reconstruction for stage iv flatfoot deformity. Foot Ankle Int 2011;32:21–30.
26. Raikin SM. Stage VI: massive osteochondral defects of the talus. Foot Ankle Clin 2004;9:737–44, vi.
27. Goldner J. Surgical treatment of the paralytic foot. Operative orthopedics. Philadelphia: J.B. Lippincott Company; 1988. p. 1799–810.
28. Mccormack AP, Ching RP, Sangeorzan BJ. Biomechanics of procedures used in adult flatfoot deformity. Foot Ankle Clin 2001;6:15–23, v.
29. Papa JA, Myerson MS. Pantalar and tibiotalocalcaneal arthrodesis for post-traumatic osteoarthrosis of the ankle and hindfoot. J Bone Joint Surg Am 1992; 74:1042–9.
30. Barg A, Knupp M, Henninger HB, et al. Total ankle replacement using Hintegra, an unconstrained, three-component system: surgical technique and pitfalls. Foot Ankle Clin 2012;17:607–35.
31. Bluman EM, Chiodo CP. Valgus ankle deformity and arthritis. Foot Ankle Clin 2008;13:443–70, ix.
32. Lee MS. Medial approach to the severe valgus foot. Clin Podiatr Med Surg 2007; 24:735–44, ix.
33. Bennett GL, Graham CE, Mauldin DM. Triple arthrodesis in adults. Foot Ankle 1991;12:138–43.
34. Pell RF, Myerson MS, Schon LC. Clinical outcome after primary triple arthrodesis. J Bone Joint Surg Am 2000;82:47–57.
35. Graves SC, Mann RA, Graves KO. Triple arthrodesis in older adults. Results after long-term follow-up. J Bone Joint Surg Am 1993;75:355–62.

36. Resnick RB, Jahss MH, Choueka J, et al. Deltoid ligament forces after tibialis posterior tendon rupture: effects of triple arthrodesis and calcaneal displacement osteotomies. Foot Ankle Int 1995;16:14–20.

37. Hyer CF, Galli MM, Scott RT, et al. Ankle valgus after hindfoot arthrodesis: a radiographic and chart comparison of the medial double and triple arthrodeses. J Foot Ankle Surg 2014;53(1):55–8.

Index

Note: Page numbers of article titles are in **boldface** type.

A

Clin Podiatr Med Surg 31 (2014) 455–460
http://dx.doi.org/10.1016/S0891-8422(14)00043-3
0891-8422/14/$ – see front matter © 2014 Elsevier Inc. All rights reserved.
podiatric.theclinics.com

Moving?

Make sure your subscription moves with you!

To notify us of your new address, find your **Clinics Account Number** (located on your mailing label above your name), and contact customer service at:

Email: journalscustomerservice-usa@elsevier.com

800-654-2452 (subscribers in the U.S. & Canada)
314-447-8871 (subscribers outside of the U.S. & Canada)

Fax number: 314-447-8029

Elsevier Health Sciences Division
Subscription Customer Service
3251 Riverport Lane
Maryland Heights, MO 63043

*To ensure uninterrupted delivery of your subscription, please notify us at least 4 weeks in advance of move.

Printed and bound by CPI Group (UK) Ltd, Croydon, CR0 4YY

03/10/2024

01040489-0014